Familial Chylomicronemia Syndrome

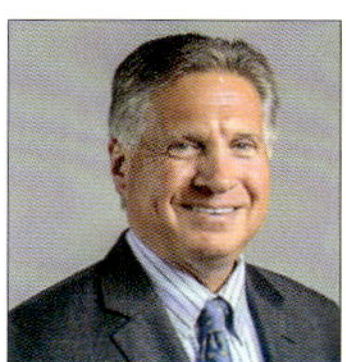

Michael H Davidson MD FACC FACP FNLA
Clinical Professor and Director of Preventive Cardiology
The University of Chicago Medicine
Chicago, Illinois, USA

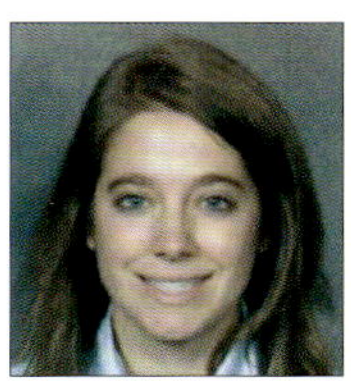

Lane Benes MD
Cardiologist, Evergreen Health
Kirkland, Washington, USA

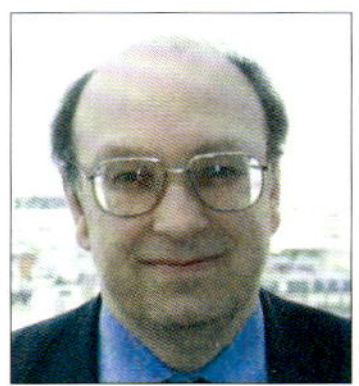

Anthony S Wierzbicki MD PhD
Consultant in Metabolic Medicine/Chemical Pathology
Professor in Cardiometabolic Disease
Guy's and St Thomas' Hospitals (King's College London)
London, UK

With thanks to **Professor Erik Stroes** MD PhD, Department of Vascular Medicine, Academic Medical Center, Amsterdam, The Netherlands, for his thorough review of this resource.

Declaration of Independence
This book is as balanced and as practical as we can make it.
Ideas for improvement are always welcome: fastfacts@karger.com

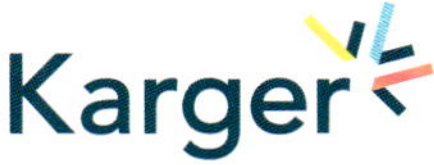

Fast Facts: Familial Chylomicronemia Syndrome
First published 2022

S. Karger Publishers Ltd, Elizabeth House, Queen Street, Abingdon,
Oxford OX14 3LN, UK
Tel: +44 (0)1235 523233

Book orders can be placed by telephone or email, or via the website.
Please telephone +41 61 306 1440 or email orders@karger.com
To order via the website, please go to karger.com

Fast Facts is a trademark of S. Karger Publishers Ltd.

A CIP record for this title is available from the British Library.

ISBN: 978-3-318-06984-6

Davidson MH (Michael)
Fast Facts: Familial Chylomicronemia Syndrome/
Michael H Davidson, Lane Benes, Anthony S Wierzbicki

Writing support for chapters 2 and 4 in the development of this publication
was provided by Andrea Gwosdow PhD, Gwosdow Associate Science
Consultants, LLC, Arlington, MA, USA.

Medical illustrations by Annamaria Dutto, Beverley, Yorkshire, UK.
Typesetting by Amnet, Chennai, India.
Printed in the UK with Xpedient Print.

This edition has been supported by an independent educational grant
from Akcea Therapeutics.

List of abbreviations

ANGPTL3: angiopoietin-like protein 3

Apo: apolipoprotein

ASO: antisense oligonucleotide

CVD: cardiovascular disease

FCS: familial chylomicronemia syndrome

FFA: free fatty acid

GPI-HBP1: glycosyl phosphatidylinositol-anchored high-density lipoprotein-binding protein 1

HDL: high-density lipoprotein

IDL: intermediate-density lipoprotein

LDL: low-density lipoprotein

LMF1: lipase maturation factor 1

LPL: lipoprotein lipase

LPLD: lipoprotein lipase deficiency

MCS: multifactorial chylomicronemia syndrome

OLE: open-label extension (study)

pCH: polygenic combined hyperlipidemia

TC: total cholesterol

TG: triglyceride

VLDL: very-low-density lipoprotein

Introduction

Familial chylomicronemia syndrome (FCS) is an ultra-rare genetic disorder characterized by the abnormal build-up of chylomicrons, the largest type of lipoprotein, which transport dietary fat from the gut to the rest of the body. Patients with FCS often experience severe symptoms, the most feared of which is acute, potentially life-threatening, pancreatitis. This resource is intended to raise awareness of FCS among all members of the healthcare team who come into contact with patients with FCS, with the aim of earlier diagnosis and management, thus preventing some of the more devastating physical, neurological and cognitive symptoms of the disorder.

FCS is not an easy disorder to manage and requires specialist input to deliver the best results. Patients must follow an extremely restricted low-fat diet, which takes an extraordinary amount of meal planning, and makes social eating an extra challenge. Even minor deviations from the diet can result in large fluctuations in serum triglyceride levels that increase the risk of acute and recurrent pancreatitis. It is therefore unsurprising that patients report anxiety, fear and worry about food and eating, the physical complications that accompany the disorder and their overall health. Standard lipid-lowering medications, including statins, fibrates and fish oils, have minimal to no effect in patients with FCS. Conversely, several therapeutic options are in development and one, volanesorsen, an antisense therapy to apolipoprotein C-III, is now licensed in Europe.

This resource offers the latest information on FCS for all members of the healthcare team, including, but not limited to, lipidologists, pancreatologists, primary care providers, dietitians, psychologists and social workers, all of whom are incredibly important in the support they provide for patients with this challenging disorder.

Terminology

Familial chylomicronemia syndrome (FCS) is an ultra-rare yet devastating autosomal recessive genetic disorder of impaired chylomicron clearance, which causes severe hypertriglyceridemia (>10 mmol/L [880 mg/dL]). The estimated prevalence of FCS is 1–10 cases per million people, affecting 3–5000 people globally.[1] Levels of serum triglycerides (TGs) are often high enough to cause acute pancreatitis, which is the most feared complication of FCS. Other names sometimes used to describe FCS are lipoprotein lipase deficiency (LPLD), familial hyperlipidemia, familial hypertriglyceridemia, familial hyperchylomicronemia and Fredrickson hyperlipoproteinemia type I (see below).

FCS versus MCS. Chylomicronemia can be monogenic or polygenic (multifactorial). FCS is the monogenic form of the disease, resulting from a loss-of-function gene mutation, and represents around 1–3% of all cases of chylomicronemia. Most cases are due to multifactorial chylomicronemia syndrome (MCS), which is most commonly polygenic in nature (see Genetics, page 12).[2] There is a large overlap between the FCS and MCS phenotypes, which can affect diagnosis and management.

Lipoproteins transport lipids from sites of synthesis to sites of use around the body. There are four major types: chylomicrons, very-low-density lipoprotein (VLDL), low-density lipoprotein (LDL) and high-density lipoprotein (HDL). Both chylomicrons and VLDL are rich in dietary TGs.

Chylomicrons are produced by enterocytes in the small intestine in response to intestinal fat absorption, and transport lipids from the gut to the rest of the body. They are predominantly composed of TGs (at least 85%), along with small proportions of phospholipids, cholesterol and proteins, of which apolipoprotein (apo) B-48 is specific to these

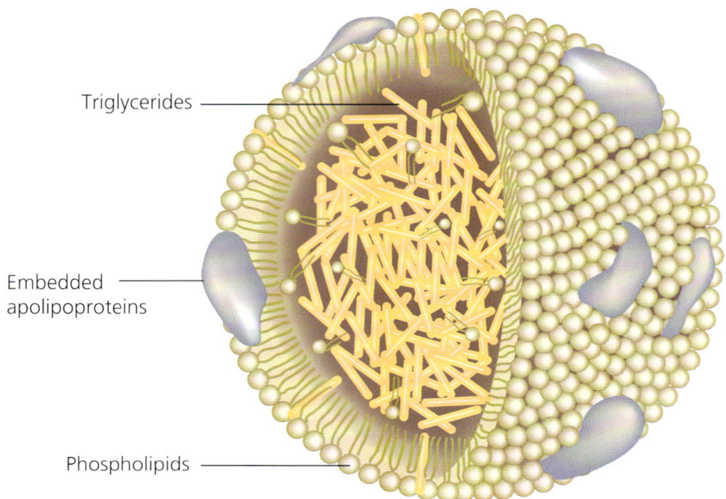

Figure 1.1 Schematic representation of a chylomicron, showing the primary constituents of insoluble triglycerides, packaged within an outer layer of phospholipids and specific apolipoproteins. Triglycerides circulate in the plasma in this form, from sites of synthesis or absorption to sites of use.

particles (Figure 1.1). In contrast, VLDL, which contains apo B-100, is produced in the liver using endogenous substrates.

Lipoprotein lipase (LPL) is a water-soluble enzyme that is synthesized and secreted by adipocytes and myocytes, respectively, and then transported to the capillary endothelial surface of peripheral tissues. Here, it removes TGs from chylomicrons and VLDL as well as other TG-carrying lipoproteins on the luminal side of the capillary endothelium (see Pathophysiology, page 14).

Lipoprotein lipase deficiency and FCS are sometimes incorrectly thought to be synonymous terms. In fact, LPLD is the most common and well-known cause of FCS, but it is only one of many variant genotypes that can yield the FCS phenotype. LPLD can lead to FCS by homozygous, compound heterozygous or double heterozygous loss of *LPL* function; 80–90% of patients with monogenic chylomicronemia have bi-allelic mutations in the *LPL* gene.[2] In addition, other genetic variants can be involved in chylomicron metabolism (that is, MCS; see Genetics, page 12).

Fredrickson hyperlipoproteinemias are classified according to the pattern of lipoprotein abnormality (Table 1.1).[3] Types I and V are often discussed together, as both can lead to TG-induced pancreatitis and share some management strategies.

Fredrickson hyperlipoproteinemia type I is synonymous with FCS. Specifically, it is a genetic disorder leading to impaired chylomicron clearance with resultant severe hypertriglyceridemia due to hyperchylomicronemia. This is the correct classification if genetic testing is positive for pathogenic variants of LPL or its cofactors.

TABLE 1.1

Fredrickson classification of lipid disorders

Fredrickson hyper-lipoproteinemia	Elevated lipoprotein(s)	Serum lipid pattern/ typical values
Type I	Chylomicrons	Elevated TGs TG >23 mmol/L (>2000 mg/dL)
Type IIa	LDL	Elevated cholesterol TC >5 mmol/L (>200 mg/dL)
Type IIb	LDL, VLDL	Elevated TGs and cholesterol TG >2.3 mmol/L (>200 mg/dL) TC >5 mmol/L (>200 mg/dL)
Type III	IDL, chylomicron remnants	Elevated TGs and cholesterol TC = TG
Type IV	VLDL	Elevated TGs TG >8.5 mmol/L (>750 mg/dL)
Type V	Chylomicrons, VLDL	Elevated TGs and TC TG >8.5 mmol/L (>750 mg/dL) TC >8 mmol/L (>300 mg/dL)

IDL, intermediate-density lipoprotein; TC, total cholesterol.

Fredrickson hyperlipoproteinemia type V is a hyperlipoproteinemia characterized by both elevated chylomicrons and VLDL. It is largely due to increased VLDL production, but often includes a component of decreased VLDL metabolism. In essence, a 'back-up' of TG-rich lipoprotein metabolism leads to hyperchylomicronemia that persists after the postprandial period. The etiology and clinical manifestations of type V are typically more varied than that of type I. Some consider type V to be a progression from type IV, in which there is isolated elevation of VLDL, or an extension of type I in those prone to increased VLDL production in addition to the genetic abnormalities leading to the hyperchylomicronemia. Acquired causes/contributors to increased VLDL levels, such as insulin resistance, obesity, excessive alcohol intake or certain medications, are common. Clinically, type V is less aggressive for any given level of hypertriglyceridemia than type I.

Genetics

***LPL* and other monogenic mutations.** FCS was first recognized in 1932 when it was diagnosed in three siblings who were found to have a deficiency of LPL. The results of studies attributed the condition to a genetic deficiency.[4] It was originally thought to be a monogenic autosomal recessive genetic disorder. Indeed, mutations in *LPL* account for more than 90% of cases,[5] which explains why the terms FCS and LPLD are often incorrectly used interchangeably (see Terminology above). There are over 100 known variants of *LPL* mutation,[6] with more yet to be discovered. Other monogenic mutations affect genes that encode co-factors of LPL, including:
- apo A-V, encoded by *APOA5*
- glycosylphosphatidylinositol-anchored high-density lipoprotein-binding protein 1 (GPI-HBP1), encoded by *GPIHBP1*
- apo C-II, encoded by *APOC2*
- lipase maturation factor 1 (LMF1), encoded by *LMF1*.

Mutations in *APOA5*, *GPIHBP1* and *APOC2* are the most common causes of monogenic FCS after *LPL*.[5,7,8] Mutations in *LMF1* are rare; only a few families have been identified with FCS caused by mutations of this gene.[5] Several mutations have been identified for each gene. The mutations of *LPL* and the genes encoding its co-factors include missense, frameshift and nonsense mutations.

Most of these autosomal recessive genotypes are compound heterozygotes, meaning that there is a different LPL variant on each gene locus, both of which impair LPL function. At this time it is thought that only homozygous, compound or double heterozygous mutations of LPL, or one of its four co-factors, leads to monogenic FCS; however, it is conceivable that homozygous or compound heterozygous mutations of other proteins involved in TG-rich lipoprotein metabolism may cause FCS as well.

Monogenic forms of FCS are equally distributed among males and females. Higher frequencies of LPLD are found in some populations, such as French Canadians, which is believed to be due to a founder effect. This has not been observed in mutations leading to deficiencies of LPL's co-factors, which have only been found in a small number of families.

Multifactorial chylomicronemia syndrome. Chylomicronemia may also be polygenic. Although there is often a homozygous, compound or double heterozygous mutation for LPLD in one of the five genes discussed above (*LPL*, *APOA5*, *GPIHBP1*, *APOC2*, *LMF1*), many cases are associated with polymorphic variants in a panel of genes associated with hypertriglyceridemia.[9] This suggests the presence of one or more additional gene variants that have yet to be identified or are not tested for in the standard five-gene panel for FCS.

For example, those with a polygenic etiology may also have an abnormal gain-of-function *APOC3* variant. Apo C-III is an inhibitor of LPL, therefore gain-of-function mutations, leading to enhanced activity/affinity for LPL, increase LPL inhibition. Researchers have shown that mice with increased *APOC3* expression have hypertriglyceridemia, while those with a null mutation have greatly reduced TG levels.[10,11]

A large number of polygenic combinations capable of causing the MCS phenotype are likely to exist, but a genetic risk score has been devised for the condition.[12]

The apparently similar phenotype of MCS means that FCS may be missed or undiagnosed. Many patients with FCS experience recurrent episodes of acute pancreatitis before the diagnosis is made. Lack of disease awareness on the part of physicians in emergency medicine, primary care and gastroenterology is a key barrier to FCS diagnosis, leading to a low rate of appropriate referrals and follow-up.

Other potential genetic etiologies. While new mutations in the five genes discussed above continue to be discovered, it is anticipated that loss-of function variants in other genes involved in TG hydrolysis will be identified as well. This could reclassify some forms of MCS as monogenic FCS. In particular, there are likely to be other key proteins involved in LPL translocation to the endothelial cell surface, factors involved in fatty acid oxidation (for example, cAMP responsive element-binding protein 3-like 3 [CREB3L3])[13] and, potentially, other co-factors or inhibitors found on the lipoprotein particle surface (see Pathophysiology below).

Non-genetic factors

Acquired deficiencies of LPL and its co-factors occur in the setting of autoimmune-mediated inhibitors of these proteins. In particular, antibodies that inhibit LPL, apo C-II and GPI-HBP1 have been identified.[14–16] Acquired causes of chylomicronemia are rare and should be managed differently from genetic causes: treatment should first be targeted at the underlying autoimmune dysfunction if possible.

Pathophysiology

Normal physiology. Soon after the consumption of a lipid-containing meal, the lipids are emulsified and digested by bile salts and pancreatic lipase. Free fatty acids (FFAs), cholesterol and other products of digestion are absorbed by the small intestine's enterocytes. The enterocytes resynthesize these products into TGs and package them into chylomicrons. TGs make up 85–92% of the chylomicron particle, with the rest comprising phospholipids, cholesterol and proteins (see Figure 1.1). The chylomicrons then enter the lacteals (small early precursors to the robust lymphatic vessels), before draining into the larger lymphatic vessels that eventually lead to the thoracic duct. From the thoracic duct, chylomicrons enter the general circulation close to the superior vena cava.

Once in the serum, chylomicrons circulate to peripheral tissues where they are initially metabolized by LPL on the endothelial surface of capillaries. There is a higher density of LPL in the capillary beds of adipose, cardiac and skeletal muscle tissues. LPL hydrolyzes the TG in the chylomicron, resulting in the release of two FFAs and monoglyceride from each TG. The FFAs are then stored or used by peripheral tissues for fuel or lipid synthesis. Parallel to this enzymatic process, proteins and other components from the chylomicron transfer to HDL-cholesterol and a chylomicron remnant remains in place of the chylomicron.

The same process occurs when LPL encounters a VLDL particle. Unlike chylomicrons, which are produced from exogenous substrates absorbed by the enterocyte, VLDL is produced by hepatocytes using mostly endogenous substrates. Hepatic TGs come from the uptake of serum FFAs, de novo hepatic lipogenesis, the recycling of TGs from the uptake of serum lipoproteins, and dietary FFAs that were not incorporated into chylomicrons and instead entered the portal vein.

When VLDL's TG component is hydrolyzed by LPL, an intermediate-density lipoprotein (IDL)-cholesterol particle remains, which eventually becomes LDL-cholesterol and is removed from the serum by the liver (Figure 1.2).

Lipoprotein lipase deficiency. Mutations of *LPL* (see Genetics, above) can lead to protein underproduction and/or transcription of an abnormal protein with a reduced ability to hydrolyze TGs. When this occurs, the TGs carried by TG-rich lipoproteins are not hydrolyzed into FFAs; instead, the TGs remain stuck on the lipoprotein, preventing structural change and further metabolism of the lipoprotein. This most greatly impacts chylomicrons, the serum levels of which fluctuate more widely than other lipoproteins under normal conditions. Normally, chylomicrons are metabolized within a few hours after a meal but in patients with LPLD they persist.

LMF1 deficiency. LPL is synthesized as an inactive monomer by the rough endoplasmic reticulum within endothelial cells located primarily in adipose, cardiac and skeletal muscle tissues.[14] LMF1 dimerizes and activates several lipases, including LPL (Figure 1.3).[17] The activated LPL is then transported to the endothelial cell surface, complexed with heparan sulfate proteoglycans.[14]

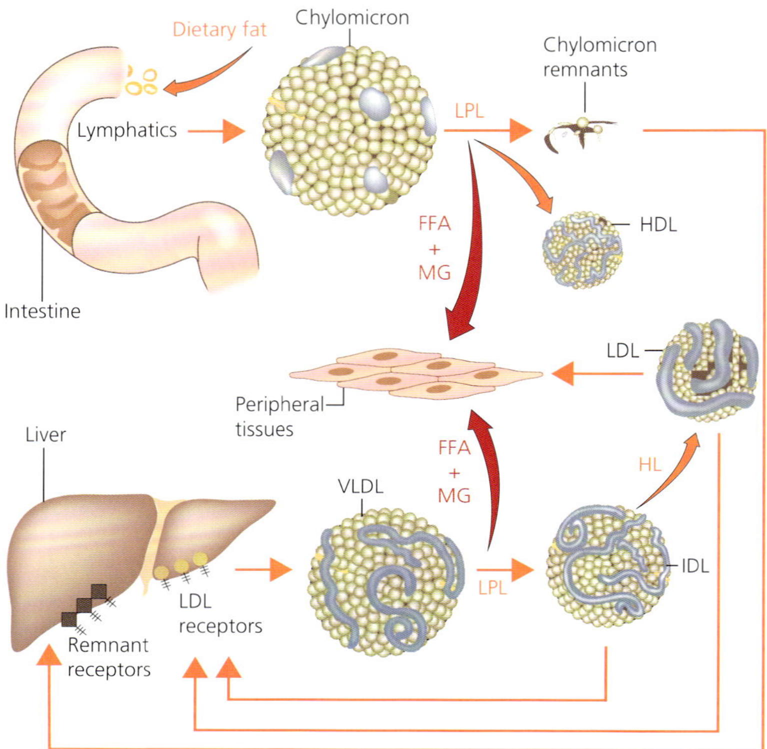

Figure 1.2 Dietary lipids are absorbed in the small intestine, packaged into chylomicrons and secreted into lymph just 1 hour after consumption. Once in circulation, chylomicrons are hydrolyzed by LPL, releasing FFAs and monoglyceride (MG), which are utilized in the peripheral tissues. Low-density components of the chylomicron are taken up by HDL, leaving chylomicron remnants that are removed from circulation by the liver. Hepatically derived VLDL follows the same catabolic pathway through LPL as chylomicrons, with the release of FFA and MG, which are utilized in the peripheral tissues. After hydrolysis, the VLDL remnant lipoprotein, called IDL, is further delipidated by hepatic lipase (HL) to LDL, which is taken up by the liver or peripheral tissues. Excess LDL may be deposited in the vessel wall, causing atherosclerosis.

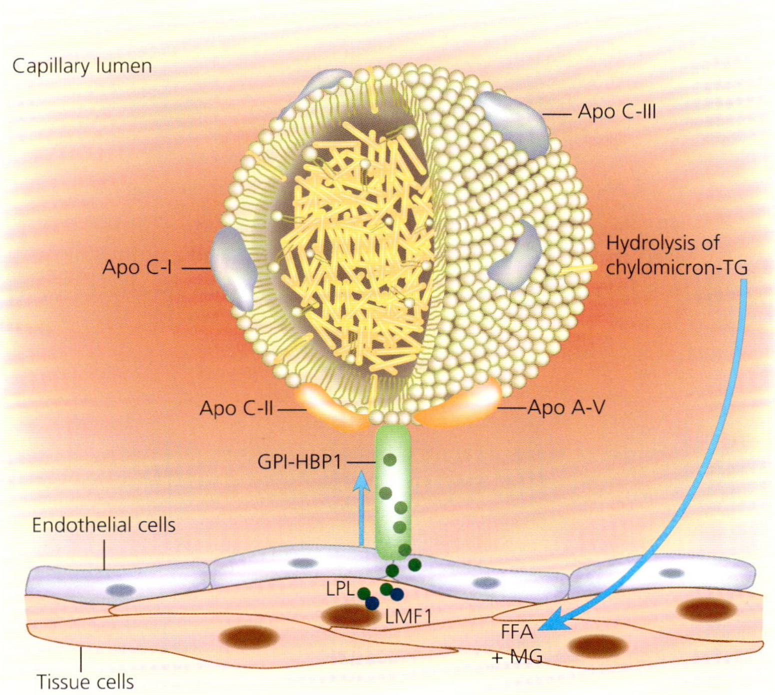

Figure 1.3 The mechanism of action of LPL is dependent on multiple regulators, both positive and negative. LMF1 is responsible for the dimerization and activation of LPL. LPL then binds to GPI-HBP1 and is transported from peripheral tissue cells to the endothelial cell surface of the capillary lumen, where apo C-II is an essential co-factor for LPL activation and apo A-V enhances LPL activity by stabilizing the LPL–apo C-II complex. In contrast, apo C-I and apo C-III inhibit LPL activity. MG, monoglyceride.

In LMF1 deficiency, normal LPL is produced but remains in an inactive form within the endothelial cell. In effect, this causes LPLD within capillary beds. The lack of TG-rich lipoprotein hydrolysis results in severe hypertriglyceridemia.

LMF1 helps activate other lipases as well, and severe deficiency of these other lipases will also impair TG hydrolysis. Mutations of *LMF1* leading to greater deficiency can cause lipodystrophy, most likely because of its global effect on the various lipases.[18]

GPI-HBP1 deficiency. GPI-HBP1 is needed to help translocate LPL to the endothelial cell surface (see Figure 1.3).[19] It also enhances lipolysis by helping anchor chylomicrons to the endothelial surface. The *GPIHBP1* mutations identified to date show loss of LPL-binding ability.[19] This results in increased LPL production and accumulation in the subendothelial space, since it is unable to be translocated to the capillary lumen. Mutations of *LPL* that alter the GPI-HBP1 binding site yield a similar result.[20]

Apolipoprotein C-II deficiency. Apo C-II is primarily produced in the liver in response to several factors, including serum TG levels. Smaller amounts are produced in other tissues. Regulation of intestinal apo C-II production is greatly affected by dietary lipid consumption. Apo C-II is incorporated onto the surface of lipoproteins, including VLDL and chylomicrons. It facilitates the binding of LPL and TG and the hydrolysis that ensues (see Figure 1.3). As the chylomicron's TG is hydrolyzed, its density and surface pressure increases, which eventually leads to displacement of LPL and apo C-II.[21] Some of the known *APOC2* mutations lead to an inability to transcribe apo C-II, or result in the production of apo C-II with decreased LPL binding and therefore reduced TG hydrolysis.[17,22]

Apolipoprotein A-V deficiency. Apo A-V's mechanisms of action have been the least well elucidated since its discovery in 2001.[23] It is produced in the liver and secreted into the plasma at relatively low concentrations compared to other lipoproteins. It is found on the surface of lipoproteins, mainly chylomicrons, VLDL and HDL (see Figure 1.3). Identified mechanisms of action include promotion of TG hydrolysis via either direct or indirect effects on LPL and enhanced lipoprotein uptake by lipoprotein receptors.[24] A proposed example of indirect modification of LPL activity would be alteration of apo C-III activity by reducing its inhibitory effect on LPL. More recently, it has been proposed that apo A-V enhances the anchoring of TG-rich lipoprotein to heparan sulfate proteoglycans, allowing interaction between LPL and other apolipoproteins and substrates.[23]

Severity according to phenotype. People with monogenic FCS due to deficiencies of apo A-V, GPIHBP1 or LMF1 may have a less severe condition and/or are diagnosed later than those with monogenic FCS due to LPL or apo C-II deficiency.[5] This is likely to be because of some effective, albeit markedly reduced, LPL actions. For example, a study of one apo A-V mutation indicated a 40% reduction in LPL activity in vitro rather than complete loss of activity.[25] In contrast, those with LPL or apo C-II deficiency may have a complete absence of LPL activity depending on mutation type.

> **Key points – terminology, etiology and pathophysiology**
>
> - FCS is a rare disorder of impaired chylomicron clearance that causes severe hypertriglyceridemia.
> - FCS is a monogenic condition, accounting for 1–3% of all cases of chylomicronemia. The phenotype is very similar to multifactorial or polygenic forms of chylomicronemia, which can affect diagnosis and management.
> - The most common monogenic cause of FCS is LPL deficiency.
> - LPL is important in the metabolism of chylomicrons, VLDL and other TG-rich lipoproteins; LPLD or deficiency of one of its co-factors results in severe hypertriglyceridemia due to the inability to hydrolyze TG on serum lipoproteins.
> - Other mutations known to cause FCS occur in the *APOA5*, *GPIHBP*, *APOC2* and *LMF1* genes, encoding the proteins apo A-V, GPI-HBP1, apo C-II and LMF1, respectively, which are all co-factors of LPL function. Mutations in other genes are likely to exist that have yet to be discovered.

References

1. Regmi M, Rehman A. Familial hyperlipidemia type 1. *StatPearls* [Internet]. Treasure Island (FL): StatPearls Publishing, 2020.

2. Baass A, Paquette M, Bernard S, Hegele RA. Familial chylomicronemia syndrome: an under-recognized cause of severe hypertriglyceridemia. *J Intern Med* 2020;287:340–8.

3. Beaumont JL, Carlson LA, Cooper GR et al. Classification of hyperlipidaemias and hyperlipoproteinaemias. *Bull World Health Organ* 1970;43:891–915.

4. Havel RJ, Gorden RS Jr. Idiopathic hyperlipemia: metabolic studies in an affected family. *J Clin Invest* 1960;39:1777–90.

5. Brahm AJ, Hegele RA. Chylomicronaemia – current diagnosis and future therapies. *Nat Rev Endocrinol* 2015;11:352–62.

6. Chokshi N, Blumenschein SD, Ahmad Z, Garg A. Genotype-phenotype relationships in patients with type I hyperlipoproteinemia. *J Clin Lipidol* 2014;8:287–95.

7. D'Erasmo L, Di Costanzo A, Cassandra F et al. Spectrum of mutations and long-term clinical outcomes in genetic chylomicronemia syndromes. *Arterioscler Thromb Vasc Biol* 2019;39:2531–41.

8. Moulin P, Dufour R, Averna M et al. Identification and diagnosis of patients with familial chylomicronaemia syndrome (FCS): expert panel recommendations and proposal of an "FCS score". *Atherosclerosis* 2018;275:265–72.

9. Johansen CT, Wang J, Lanktree MB et al. An increased burden of common and rare lipid-associated risk alleles contributes to the phenotypic spectrum of hypertriglyceridemia. *Arterioscler Thromb Vasc Biol* 2011;31:1916–26.

10. Ito Y, Azrolan N, O'Connell A et al. Hypertriglyceridemia as a result of human apo CIII gene expression in transgenic mice. *Science* 1990;249:790–3.

11. Maeda N, Li H, Lee D et al. Targeted disruption of the apolipoprotein C-III gene in mice results in hypotriglyceridemia and protection from postprandial hypertriglyceridemia. *J Biol Chem* 1994;269:23610–16.

12. Hegele RA, Ginsberg HN, Chapman MJ et al.; European Atherosclerosis Society Consensus Panel. The polygenic nature of hypertriglyceridaemia: implications for definition, diagnosis, and management. *Lancet Diabetes Endocrinol* 2014;2:655–66.

13. Dron JS, Dilliott AA, Lawson A et al. Loss-of-function *CREB3L3* variants in patients with severe hypertriglyceridemia. *Arterioscler Thromb Vasc Biol* 2020;40:1935–41.

14. Mead JR, Irvine SA, Ramji DP. Lipoprotein lipase: structure, function, regulation, and role in disease. *J Mol Med (Berl)* 2002;80:753–69.

15. Yamamoto H, Tanaka M, Yoshiga S et al. Autoimmune hypertriglyceridemia induced by anti-apolipoprotein CII antibody. *J Clin Endocrinol Metab* 2014;99: 1525–30.

16. Beigneux AP, Miyashita K, Ploug M et al. Autoantibodies against GPIHBP1 as a cause of hypertriglyceridemia. *N Engl J Med* 2017;376:1647–58.

17. Wolska A, Dunbar RL, Freeman LA et al. Apolipoprotein C-II: new findings related to genetics, biochemistry, and role in triglyceride metabolism. *Atherosclerosis* 2017; 267:49–60.

18. Péterfy M. Lipase maturation factor 1: a lipase chaperone involved in lipid metabolism. *Biochim Biophys Acta* 2012;1821:790–4.

19. Davies BS, Beigneux AP, Barnes RH 2nd et al. GPIHBP1 is responsible for the entry of lipoprotein lipase into capillaries. *Cell Metab* 2010;12:42–52.

20. Gin P, Goulbourne CN, Adeyo O et al. Chylomicronemia mutations yield new insights into interactions between lipoprotein lipase and GPIHBP1. *Hum Mol Genet* 2012; 21:2961–72.

21. Meyers NL, Larsson M, Olivecrona G, Small DM. A pressure-dependent model for the regulation of lipoprotein lipase by apolipoprotein C-II. *J Biol Chem* 2015;290:18029–44.

22. Fojo SS, Brewer HB. Hypertriglyceridaemia due to genetic defects in lipoprotein lipase and apolipoprotein C-II. *J Intern Med* 1992;231:669–77.

23. Gonzales JC, Gordts PL, Foley EM, Esko JD. Apolipoproteins E and AV mediate lipoprotein clearance by hepatic proteoglycans. *J Clin Invest* 2013;123:2742–51.

24. Nilsson SK, Heeren J, Olivecrona G, Merkel M. Apolipoprotein A-V; a potent triglyceride reducer. *Atherosclerosis* 2011;219:15–21.

25. Priore Oliva C, Pisciotta L, Li Volti G et al. Inherited apolipoprotein A-V deficiency in severe hypertriglyceridemia. *Arterioscler Thromb Vasc Biol* 2005;25:411–17.

Clinical presentation

FCS is the most severe phenotype of chylomicronemia. Patients with this autosomal recessive monogenic form of the disease often manifest in childhood or early adulthood, while those with MCS may present a decade or two later. FCS is usually diagnosed in childhood or adolescence, or in people under 40 years of age.

Signs and symptoms. Not uncommonly, severe abdominal and/or back pain due to pancreatitis is the initial presentation leading to the diagnosis of FCS. The pain often radiates from the side to the back. Severe abdominal pain is often triggered by eating or drinking alcohol and may be accompanied by nausea and vomiting. The frequent, often chronic, pain and complications of pancreatitis and eventual pancreatic insufficiency cause significant morbidity. Other signs and symptoms,[1] many of which are discussed in more detail in Chapter 3, are summarized in Table 2.1.

Eruptive xanthomas are typically seen on the knees, shoulders, lateral extremities and buttocks. An examination of the visual system with fundoscopy often reveals lipemia retinalis, which is seen as whitened retinal blood vessels. However, vision is usually not impaired by this condition.

Diagnostic tests

FCS may be suspected in symptomatic patients or patients treated for pancreatitis, anyone with severe hypertriglyceridemia in whom secondary causes such as uncontrolled diabetes or alcohol misuse have been ruled out, or those with a family history of FCS.

Fasting lipid panel. Severe or recurrent episodes of abdominal pain should trigger a fasting lipid panel to measure serum TGs, total cholesterol (TC), LDL and HDL. A high fasting serum TG level of at least 10 mmol/L (880 mg/dL) in three consecutive blood

TABLE 2.1

Common signs and symptoms of FCS*

- Severe abdominal and/or back pain
- Failure to thrive
- Lipemia retinalis
- Hepatosplenomegaly
- Eruptive xanthomas
- Fatigue/malaise
- Dyspnea
- Numbness in feet or legs
- Depression
- Memory loss
- Cognitive impairment

*See Chapter 3 for more details.

samples indicates FCS. Patients with FCS also have low or normal LDL, normal HDL and a TG:TC ratio greater than 2.2 (if mmol/L units) (Table 2.2).

Refrigerator test. The hallmark of FCS is the abnormal persistence of chylomicrons after a fasting period of 12–14 hours, which appear as lactescent plasma, that is, a creamy-milky top layer in blood samples after refrigeration (Figure 2.1).[2] Overnight refrigeration of plasma can distinguish Fredrickson hyperlipoproteinemia type I and V (see page 11): type I develops a creamy top layer only, whereas type V develops both a creamy top layer and a turbid adjacent layer, indicating the presence of VLDL.

Differential diagnosis

The differential diagnosis of FCS includes other causes of hypertriglyceridemia and genetic disease (Table 2.3). This requires a complete family history.

TABLE 2.2

Biochemical characteristics of FCS

Parameter	Range
Fasting TG	>10 mmol/L (880 mg/dL)
LDL	Normal to low
HDL	Normal
TG:TC ratio	>2.2 if mmol/L units (>5 if mg/dL units)
Apo B_{100}	<1.9 µmol/L (100 mg/dL)

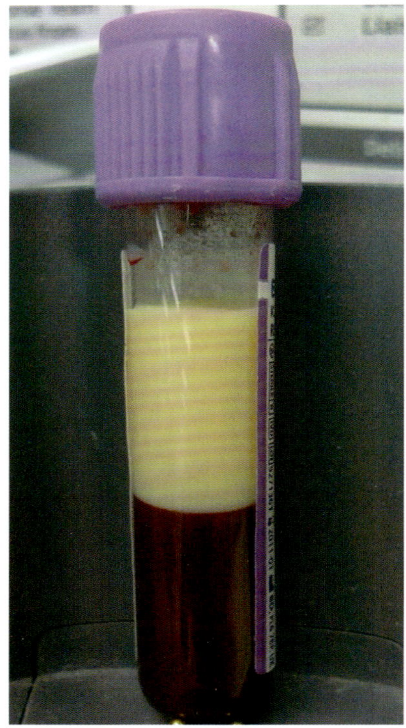

Figure 2.1 Chylomicrons have the lowest density of all lipoproteins and will float to the top of a blood sample when refrigerated overnight, forming a cream-like layer.

TABLE 2.3

Other causes of severe hypertriglyceridemia

- Dietary issues (extreme excess of carbohydrate or refined sugar drinks)
- Diabetes mellitus (uncontrolled)
- Alcohol abuse
- Paraproteinemic disorders
- MCS
- Dysbetalipoproteinemia
- Lipodystrophy syndromes
- Physiological (third trimester of pregnancy)
- Medications (see Table 4.3, page 49)

Notes: Renal disease, nephrotic syndrome, hypothyroidism and pregnancy may cause hypertriglyceridemia on a background of a genetic triglyceridemia trait. Adapted from Burnett et al. 2017 and Stroes et al. 2017.[3,4]

As shown in Table 2.2, evaluating the levels of LDL, HDL and TG:TC is one way of differentiating FCS from other metabolic disorders. Apo B levels can differentiate FCS from polygenic combined hyperlipidemia (pCH). Patients with pCH have apo B levels greater than 2.3 μmol/L (120 mg/dL), while patients with FCS have apo B_{100} levels below 1.9 μmol/L (100 mg/dL). Dysbetalipoproteinemia can be differentiated from FCS by sequencing the gene responsible for apo E.

Lipid-lowering medications often have minimal to no effect on TG levels in patients with FCS, so a 3-month trial of a lipid-lowering drug can confirm the possibility of FCS.[4]

Other tests that may be helpful in distinguishing FCS from other metabolic disorders include chylomicron determination, fasting blood glucose or glycated hemoglobin levels, urinalysis, liver function tests and biopsy of eruptive xanthomas.

Confirmation of FCS diagnosis

While high serum TGs are always seen in FCS, one or more of the following symptoms is also required for the diagnosis (Figure 2.2):

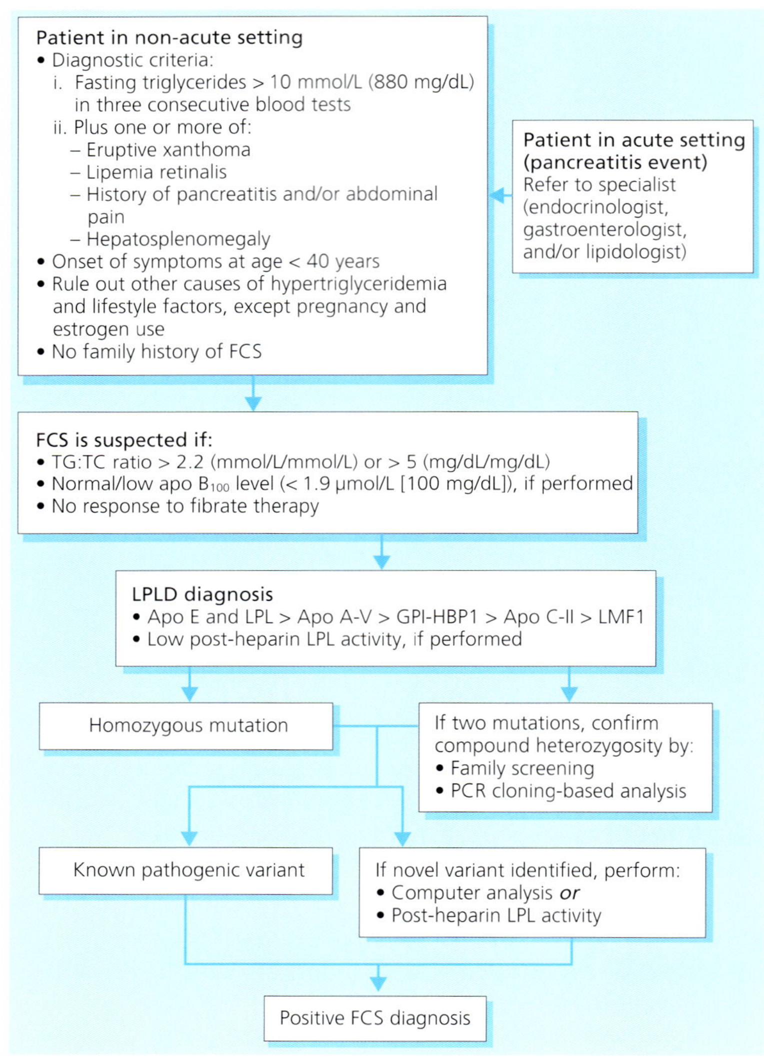

Figure 2.2 Algorithm for a positive diagnosis of FCS. Adapted from Davidson et al. 2017 and Stroes et al. 2017.[1,4]

- eruptive xanthomas
- lipemia retinalis
- recurrent abdominal pain
- pancreatitis
- hepatosplenomegaly.

Genetic testing. A definitive diagnosis of monogenic FCS is made by full gene sequencing of the *LPL* gene and the genes that enable LPL to function (see Figure 2.2).[3] The associated genes are those that encode apo A-V (*APOA5*), GPI-HBP1 (*GPIHBP1*), apo C-II (*APOC2*) and LMF1 (*LMF1*).[4,5] In monogenic FCS, genetic testing will show homozygous or compound or double heterozygous loss-of-function variants in *LPL* or one of the associated genes.

In patients with MCS, only one or no alleles with a loss-of-function variant may be identified. Their phenotype, however, may still be the same or very similar to those with confirmed monogenic FCS; this may be explained by the presence of yet-to-be discovered mutations in these or other enzymes involved in chylomicron metabolism. As the name implies, those with MCS may have several variants, which alone may not be as devastating but together culminate in a more severe phenotype.

Genetic mutations are assessed by comparison with curated lists of pathogenic variants (mutations) known to cause FCS.[6,7] This genetic information determines which protein(s) are not functioning properly and provides information on the nature of the metabolic disorder. If more than one mutation is present, transcriptome (messenger RNA) analysis or family screening is used to assess chromosome phase, simple or compound heterozygosity.[4]

Genetic testing may reveal a variant of unknown significance, especially in genes where few affected cases have been described. If this occurs, the enzyme activity levels of LPL should be measured, as patients with mutations in the *LPL* gene or related genes have reduced or low levels of LPL activity (see Chapter 1).

Diagnostic scoring system

Taking all the above information into account, a scoring system that utilizes clinical, laboratory and genetic criteria has been developed to diagnose FCS (Table 2.4).[8]

TABLE 2.4

FCS scoring system

- Fasting TGs >10 mmol/L (880 mg/dL) for 3 consecutive blood analyses at least 1 month apart (+5)
  - Fasting TGs >20 mmol/L (1755 mg/dL) at least once (+1)
- Previous TGs <2 mmol/L (–5)
- No secondary factors (except pregnancy and ethinylestradiol) (+2)
- History of pancreatitis (+1)
- Unexplained recurrent abdominal pain (+1)
- No history of familial combined hyperlipidemia (+1)
- No response (TG decrease <20%) to hypolipidemic treatment (+1)
- Onset of symptoms at age:
  <40 years (+1)
  <20 years (+2)
  <10 years (+3)

FCS score	
≥10	FCS very likely
≤9	FCS unlikely
≤8	FCS very unlikely

Reproduced from Moulin et al. 2018,[8] with permission from Elsevier.

Key points – diagnosis

- The most common initial presentation of FCS is severe or recurring abdominal pain due to acute, chronic or recurrent pancreatitis.
- FCS should be suspected if fasting serum TG levels are greater than 10 mmol/L (880 mg/dL) in three consecutive blood samples.
- In addition to high TG levels, one or more of the following symptoms must be present: eruptive xanthomas, lipemia retinalis, recurrent abdominal pain, pancreatitis and/or hepatosplenomegaly. Genetic confirmation is also needed.
- FCS must be distinguished from other causes of hypertriglyceridemia. Diagnostic tests that will help distinguish FCS from other metabolic disorders include a complete lipid panel, chylomicron determination, fasting blood glucose level or glycated hemoglobin, liver function tests, urinalysis and (if necessary) biopsy of eruptive xanthomas.
- The gold standard for confirming the diagnosis of monogenic FCS is sequencing of the *LPL* gene along with other genes that enable LPL to function: *APOA5*, *GPIHBP1*, *APOC2* and *LMF1*.
- MCS, in which there is only one or no alleles with a loss-of-function mutation, has recently been recognized. Patients with MCS still demonstrate a phenotype that overlaps with FCS, after excluding secondary hypertriglyceridemia.
- A scoring system for the diagnosis of FCS that utilizes clinical, laboratory and genetic criteria is now available.

References

1. Davidson M, Stevenson M, Hsieh A et al. The burden of familial chylomicronemia syndrome: interim results from the IN-FOCUS study. *Expert Rev Cardiovasc Ther* 2017; 15:415–23.

2. Tremblay K, Méthot J, Brisson D, Gaudet D. Etiology and risk of lactescent plasma and severe hypertriglyceridemia. *J Clin Lipidol* 2011;5:37–44.

3. Burnett JR, Hooper AJ, Hegele RA. Familial lipoprotein lipase deficiency. In: Adam MP, Ardinger HH, Pagon RA, eds. *GeneReviews®* [Internet]. Seattle (WA): University of Washington, Seattle; 1993–2018. 1999 Oct 12 (updated 22 June 2017).

4. Stroes E, Moulin P, Parhofer KG et al. Diagnostic algorithm for familial chylomicronemia syndrome. *Atheroscler Suppl* 2017;23:1–7.

5. Brahm AJ, Hegele R. Chylomicronaemia – current diagnosis and future therapies. *Nat Rev Endocrinol* 2015;11:352–62.

6. Fu J, Kwok S, Sinai L et al. Western database of lipid variants (WDLV): a catalogue of genetic variants in monogenic dyslipidemias. *Can J Cardiol* 2013;29:934–9.

7. Rodrigues R, Artieda M, Tejedor D et al. Pathogenic classification of LPL gene variants reported to be associated with LPL deficiency. *J Clin Lipidol* 2016;10:394–409.

8. Moulin P, Dufour R, Averna M et al. Identification and diagnosis of patients with familial chylomicronaemia syndrome (FCS): expert panel recommendations and proposal of an "FCS score". *Atherosclerosis* 2018;275:265–72.

Severity

As discussed in Chapter 1, there are several genotypes of FCS and therefore the severity of the phenotype can vary. Within the different monogenic forms of the disorder, with homozygous or compound heterozygous loss of LPL function, the large number of *LPL* mutations means that the magnitude of LPLD varies. Patients with more devastating mutations may present in childhood or early adulthood with skin manifestations or acute pancreatitis, while others may not be diagnosed until the third or fourth decade of life, with severe hypertriglyceridemia only being discovered on a routine screening lipid panel.

In general, those with MCS tend to present later, since they do not have an obvious homozygous or compound heterozygous deficiency in LPL or one of its co-factors. This enables the lipoprotein metabolism cascades to partially compensate for the presumably heterozygous deficiencies. Some patients with MCS may worsen after developing a secondary cause of hypertriglyceridemia, such as diabetes or certain medication use, leading to their initial presentation. This can include elevations of VLDL TGs in addition to the hyperchylomicronemia. Some experts reclassify such patients from Fredrickson hyperlipoproteinemia type I to type V; this is reasonable as long as it is understood that the predominant underlying pathophysiology causing the hyperchylomicronemia is unchanged. These patients still benefit from the same management approach, with the possible addition of treatment targeting the secondary cause of worsening hypertriglyceridemia, if applicable.

Complications of FCS due to the severe hypertriglyceridemia include abdominal pain secondary to pancreatitis, eruptive xanthomas, lipemia retinalis, hepatosplenomegaly and neurocognitive dysfunction. Patients also experience considerable psychological morbidity. The relationship between FCS and atherosclerotic cardiovascular disease (CVD) is not as well described as that between more common hypertriglyceridemias and atherosclerotic CVD, but what is known is discussed in this chapter.

Acute pancreatitis

Etiology and epidemiology. Severe hypertriglyceridemia is the third most common cause of acute pancreatitis after gallstones and alcohol ingestion, accounting for 1–10% of all pancreatitis episodes.[1]

TG-induced pancreatitis is generally more severe than acute pancreatitis due to other etiologies, in terms of both severity scores and clinical outcomes.[2] It is associated with a higher rate of persistent organ failure, increased admission to the intensive care unit and longer hospitalization than other etiologies of acute pancreatitis with normal TG levels,[3] and for these reasons it is the most feared complication of FCS.

A survey of 10 patients with FCS found that the total number of self-reported episodes of acute pancreatitis ranged from 6 to 60 with a median of 34 episodes.[4] These included cases managed at home as well as with medical care, with a median number of 17 hospitalizations for acute pancreatitis per patient. Of note, this sample may be subject to referral bias because of over-representation of more severe FCS phenotypes. The rate of at least one episode of pancreatitis in patients with FCS seems to be 40–60%.[5–7]

The risk of developing pancreatitis is generally thought to increase when serum TG starts to surpass 11.3 mmol/L (1000 mg/dL), and the risk increases further as serum TG levels continue to rise. Given the high morbidity and mortality associated with pancreatitis, the foremost goal of FCS treatment is to lower serum TG below 11.3 mmol/L (1000 mg/dL) to significantly lower the risk of acute pancreatitis. Further discussion of preventing and treating acute pancreatitis can be found in Chapter 4.

Clinical presentation of TG-induced acute pancreatitis is the same as that of other etiologies, and often consists of epigastric, abdominal and/or mid-back pain and nausea and vomiting. If there is a sufficiently robust inflammatory response, the patient may be hypotensive and intravascularly volume depleted due to fluid redistribution to a third space.

In addition to the development of systemic inflammatory response syndrome, other complications include necrotizing pancreatitis with or without superimposed infection, hemorrhage, pseudocyst formation, acute respiratory distress syndrome, multiorgan failure and death.[8,9] The complication rate appears to be at least as high as that of other causes of pancreatitis, although the exact rate is unclear.[2]

Pathophysiology. The mechanism behind TG-induced acute pancreatitis is not well understood. It is likely to involve the secretion of pancreatic lipase into the local vasculature, leading to extensive TG hydrolysis and FFA production, which in turn causes local damage to pancreatic cells, either directly or indirectly by the inflammatory response (Figure 3.1).[1] Ischemia of pancreatic vessels due to TG-

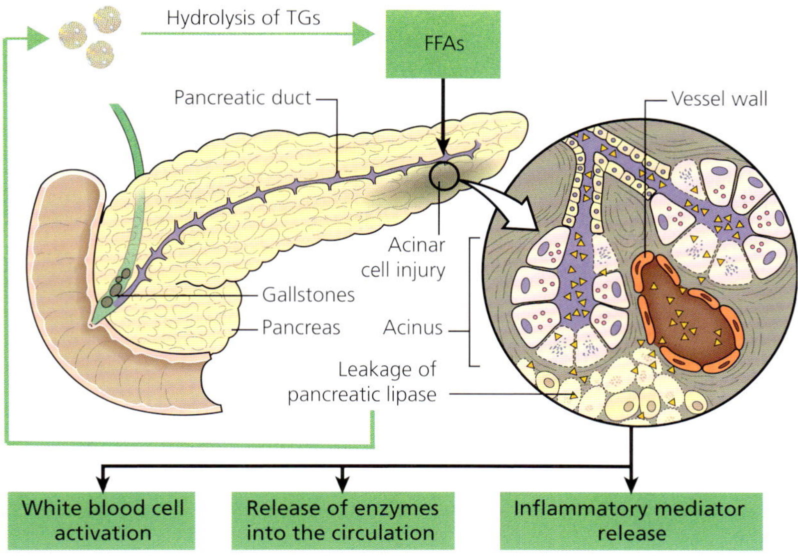

Figure 3.1 Possible pathogenesis of TG-induced acute pancreatitis. High levels of TGs may cause local damage to pancreatic acinar cells, leading to leakage of pancreatic lipase into the interstitial space and further cytotoxic injury to pancreatic cells from the increase in FFAs released from TGs. Apoptosis or necrosis of pancreatic acinar cells leads to a systemic inflammatory response syndrome, with white blood cell activity and the release of enzymes and inflammatory mediators.

induced serum viscosity or the viscosity caused by high levels of FFAs may cause or contribute to acute pancreatic injury.[1] The release of pancreatic lipase and other digestive enzymes from the damaged exocrine acinar cells leads to further pancreatic injury, and may also hydrolyze TG in surrounding adipose tissue, releasing more FFAs. If these FFAs enter the bloodstream, they further contribute to the high FFA load and are also likely to exacerbate pancreatic injury (see Figure 3.1).

Chronic pancreatitis

Frequent episodes of acute pancreatitis can lead to chronic pancreatitis, which is characterized by permanent damage of structure and/or function.[10] This may manifest as atrophy, calcification, pancreatic stones and/or ductal dilatation and strictures (Figure 3.2).[10]

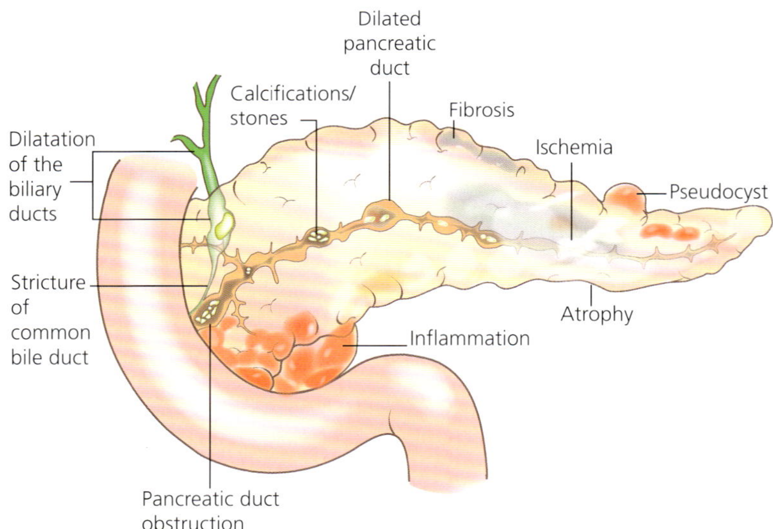

Figure 3.2 Chronic pancreatitis is a progressive inflammatory process that causes fibrosis, calcifications or stones and/or dilatation of the pancreatic duct. Complications include pseudocyst formation and pancreatic or biliary strictures.

Functional damage often includes loss of exocrine function requiring enzymatic replacement for proper meal absorption and/or loss of endocrine function leading to diabetes. Complications of chronic pancreatitis include pseudocyst formation, pancreatic or biliary strictures and increased risk of pancreatic cancer.[10] The most common symptom is chronic abdominal pain, which may lead to long-term administration of pain medication.

Eruptive xanthomas

Epidemiology and clinical presentation. Eruptive xanthomas occur in about 24% of patients with FCS.[4] They usually have an abrupt onset, presenting as multiple yellow-to-red papules of 1–5 mm in diameter (Figure 3.3).

The most common sites are the extensor surfaces of extremities and the buttocks. Eruptive xanthomas on these sites are highly correlated with severe hypertriglyceridemia, and are therefore associated with Fredrickson hyperlipoproteinemia types I and V, and to a lesser extent type IV. Tuberous and tendinous xanthomas on the other hand are characteristically observed in hypercholesterolemia, as they are manifestations of cholesterol deposition. Tuberous xanthomas are

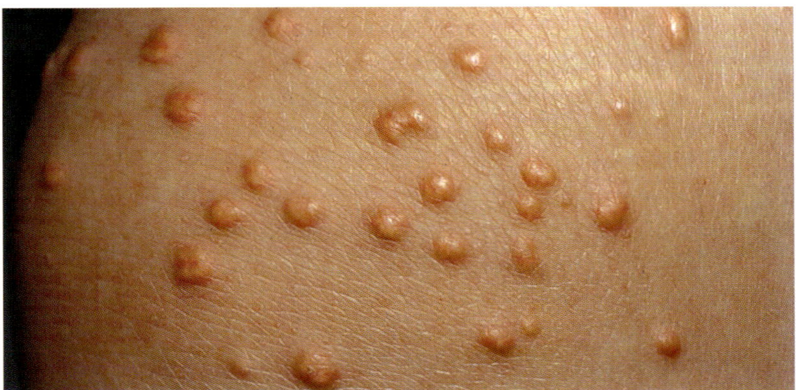

Figure 3.3 Eruptive xanthomas, presenting as multiple yellow-to-red papules of 1–5 mm in diameter on the knees of a patient with FCS. Reproduced courtesy of Gary M White MD, RegionalDerm.com.

similar to eruptive xanthomas in color and location but are larger and present either as single papules or nodules or as a cluster of papules/nodules. Of note, xanthelasmas, which are thin yellow papules or plaques found around the eyelids, are seen in patients with and without hyperlipidemia and are therefore a non specific finding.

Pathogenesis. Although the pathogenic mechanism of eruptive xanthoma development is not fully elucidated at this time, histological analysis and electron microscopy in patients with severely elevated chylomicron-TGs appear to show that the chylomicrons permeate dermal capillary walls. This leads to TG accumulation in the extracellular space, cells near the endothelium and macrophages, leading to foam-cell aggregates that manifest as an eruptive xanthoma.[11] Other inflammatory cells may be involved in the lesion. Interestingly, when serum TG is significantly reduced, the composition of the xanthoma changes: TG is removed and cholesterol esters become the predominant lipid.[11]

Long-term effects. Eruptive xanthomas are not known to be harmful, but resolution may be desired for cosmetic reasons. It is unclear if the presence of eruptive xanthomas indicates a higher risk of coronary artery disease in patients with FCS. It has been shown that in those with heterozygous familial hypercholesterolemia, the presence of tendon xanthomas (with a different pathogenesis) is associated with a threefold higher risk of CVD.[12] Xanthoma formation in hypercholesterolemia is analogous to, but not identical to, eruptive xanthomas in patients with severe hypertriglyceridemia. Therefore, the association between hypercholesterolemic xanthomatosis and CVD cannot be assumed to apply to patients with FCS with eruptive xanthomas.

Lipemia retinalis

Clinical presentation. On funduscopic examination in patients with severe hypertriglyceridemia, retinal vessels appear creamy (rather than the normal dark-red appearance) due to oversaturation of chylomicron-TG (Figure 3.4).

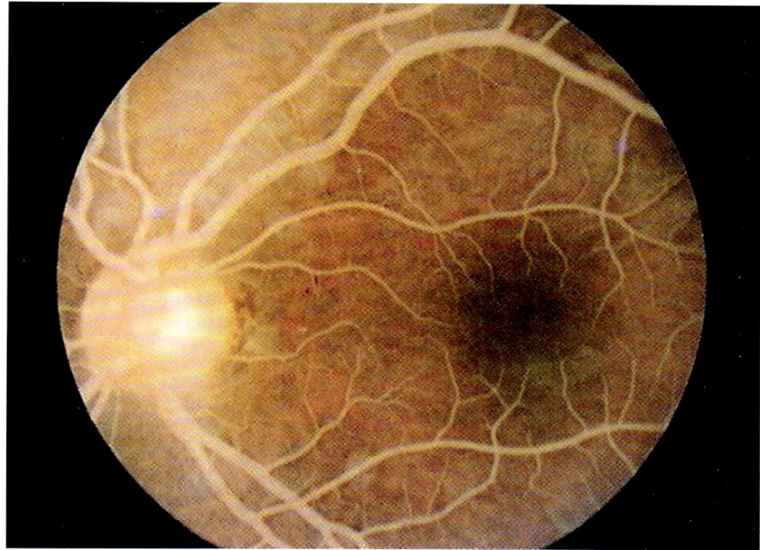

Figure 3.4 Lipemia retinalis: retinal vessels appear creamy in color, rather than dark red, due to oversaturation of chylomicron-TG. In this case, the entire background of the fundus is a milky-salmon color, which is usually observed when TG levels exceed 57 mmol/L (5000 mg/dL). Reproduced courtesy of Ted M Montgomery, optometric physician, tedmontgomery.com/the_eye/eyephotos/index.html.

Epidemiology and etiology. TG levels are usually around 28 mmol/L (2500 mg/dL) when lipemia retinalis is first observed. The periphery of the fundus is the first area to become abnormal, followed by the posterior pole when TG levels approach 40–57 mmol/L (3500–5000 mg/dL).[13] The use of ultrawide field scanning laser ophthalmoscopy may improve the detection rate by better visualizing the periphery. In addition to the change in vessel appearance, the entire background of the fundus can be lighter in color than normal and has been described as a milky-salmon color; this is usually observed when TG levels exceed 57 mmol/L (5000 mg/dL) (see Figure 3.4).[13,14]

Long-term effects. When serum TG levels are lowered, the severity of lipemia retinalis is reduced and may completely resolve. Cases in which lipemia retinalis alters vision have been reported,[15] but it is generally not thought to affect visual acuity. Whether longstanding lipemia retinalis leads to permanent ophthalmic changes is unknown.

Hepatosplenomegaly

Pathophysiology. Extravasation of chylomicron-TG from the bloodstream into hepatic and splenic tissue can lead to the development of hepatosplenomegaly. Similar to dermal xanthoma formation, engulfment by macrophages in these tissues leads to foam-cell formation; when this occurs to a significant degree, organomegaly ensues.

Epidemiology. The finding of hepatosplenomegaly is rarely the presenting abnormality that leads to a diagnosis of FCS; both sensitivity and specificity are low. However, assessing for its presence on physical examination adds minimal time and effort and is therefore worthwhile doing. In one survey of lipidologists, hepatosplenomegaly was found in 43% of patients with FCS.[7]

Long-term effects. With effective TG-lowering treatment, hepatosplenomegaly resolves in approximately 1 week. It is conceivable that longstanding hepatomegaly could lead to inflammation with resultant fibrosis. However, TG-induced cirrhosis has not been described in patients with FCS.

Psychological burden

It is unsurprising that patients with FCS experience significant psychological morbidity given the extreme challenge of adhering to a highly restrictive diet and the extent of physical complications that often accompany the disorder. The first robust survey to assess the burden of the condition and its effect on quality of life is the Investigation of Findings and Observations Captured in Burden of Illness Survey (IN-FOCUS). IN-FOCUS is an internet-based survey that was initially filled out by 60 patients with FCS in the USA; 106 patients have since been added globally.[5] Initial results from the US survey showed that 22% of participants frequently felt sad/down/blue/depressed.[5]

The international survey of 166 participants determined that the four primary contributing factors to psychological morbidity were:

- constant uncertainty about an attack of acute pancreatitis or pain (33%)
- fear/anxiety/worry about their health (23%)
- uncertainty about diet (19%)
- feeling out of control/helpless because of their FCS (17%).

In addition, 94% of respondents reported that their employment status was affected by FCS.

Neurocognitive dysfunction

Some patients with FCS may experience transient periods of neurocognitive dysfunction. To date, this has received minimal study and it is not known if there is a threshold serum TG level above which it occurs; it is likely to vary for each patient. Most data are from the global IN-FOCUS survey, which found that the most commonly experienced cognitive symptoms are difficulty concentrating (14%), impaired judgment (10%), 'brain fog' (8%) and forgetfulness (7%), all of which occurred daily or every other day. FCS-related cognitive impairment may also affect most patients' employment status, even if only occasionally. Neurocognitive dysfunction may be due to decreased energy secondary to physical symptoms and/or compromised cerebral perfusion from the hyperviscosity of severe hypertriglyceridemia.

Atherosclerotic cardiovascular disease

Whether FCS increases CVD risk is uncertain; case reports are contradictory. There is a well-established association between elevated TG-rich lipoproteins and CVD,[16] but this may not apply to patients with FCS, except possibly for those with the *APOA5* gene, which is known to be independently associated with CVD.[17] To date, studies assessing the link between hypertriglyceridemia and CVD have almost exclusively included those with a more common hypertriglyceridemia caused by VLDL-TG rather than chylomicron-TG.

The large size of chylomicrons is thought to confer less atherogenicity than other lipoproteins, and cases of patients with FCS without accelerated atherosclerosis have been reported.[18,19] This may in part be explained by the fact that patients with FCS have normal or low apo B_{100} levels; apo B_{100} has been shown to better predict CVD risk than non-HDL lipoproteins,[20] the latter being very high in FCS as a result of the severely elevated TGs. Cases demonstrating increased CVD in patients with FCS have been reported as well.[21]

More research is needed to determine whether patients with FCS are at increased CVD risk. At this time, we favor the hypothesis that FCS alone in the absence of established CVD risk factors does not lead to an increased risk. If our hypothesis is incorrect, chylomicrons may be more atherogenic than previously thought, or perhaps severe hypertriglyceridemia leads to increased inflammation, increasing the risk of atheromatous diseases. It is also unknown if there is a difference in risk between those with monogenic and polygenic FCS. The latter are more likely to have increased VLDL-TG, which may increase CVD risk.

Key points – complications

- The phenotype of FCS varies. Some genetic mutations lead to severe physical manifestations in childhood, while others may go undiagnosed until severe hypertriglyceridemia is detected on a routine screening lipid panel in the third or fourth decade of life.
- Pancreatitis, which affects about 40–60% of people with FCS, is the most worrisome complication of FCS because of the significant risk of associated complications, including death.
- Acute episodes of pancreatitis can lead to chronic pancreatitis and pancreatic insufficiency. This often includes chronic abdominal and/or back pain.
- Additional physical complications include eruptive xanthomas, lipemia retinalis and hepatosplenomegaly. Fortunately, these complications quickly improve or even resolve with effective TG-lowering treatment.
- FCS is also associated with significant psychological morbidity, and up to 20% of patients experience neurocognitive dysfunction.
- Most people with FCS report that their employment status and/or career choice have been affected by the disorder.
- It is unclear whether people with FCS are at increased risk of atherosclerotic CVD.

References

1. Valdivielso P, Ramírez-Bueno A, Ewald N. Current knowledge of hypertriglyceridemic pancreatitis. *Eur J Intern Med* 2014;25:689–94.

2. Carr RA, Rejowski BJ, Cote GA et al. Systematic review of hypertriglyceridemia-induced acute pancreatitis: a more virulent etiology? *Pancreatology* 2016; 16:469–76.

3. Nawaz H, Koutroumpakis E, Easler J et al. Elevated serum triglycerides are independently associated with persistent organ failure in acute pancreatitis. *Am J Gastroenterol* 2015;110:1497–503.

4. Gelrud A, Williams KR, Hsieh A et al. The burden of familial chylomicronemia syndrome from the patients' perspective. *Expert Rev Cardiovasc Ther* 2017;15:879–87.

5. Davidson M, Stevenson M, Hsieh A et al. The burden of familial chylomicronemia syndrome: interim results from the IN-FOCUS study. *Expert Rev Cardiovasc Ther* 2017; 15:415–23.

6. Rabacchi C, Pisciotta L, Cefalù AB et al. Spectrum of mutations of the *LPL* gene identified in Italy in patients with severe hypertriglyceridemia. *Atherosclerosis* 2015;241:79–86.

7. Gaudet D, Blom D, Bruckert E et al. Acute pancreatitis is highly prevalent and complications can be fatal in patients with familial chylomicronemia: results from a survey of lipidologists. *J Clin Lipidol* 2016;10:680–1.

8. Marshall JB. Acute pancreatitis. A review with an emphasis on new developments. *Arch Intern Med* 1993;153:1185–98.

9. Frossard JL, Steer ML, Pastor CM. Acute pancreatitis. *Lancet* 2008;371: 143–52.

10. Mitchell RM, Byrne MF, Baillie J. Pancreatitis. *Lancet* 2003;361: 1447–55.

11. Parker F, Bagdade JD, Odland GF, Bierman EL. Evidence for the chylomicron origin of lipids accumulating in diabetic eruptive xanthomas: a correlative lipid biochemical, histochemical, and electron microscopic study. *J Clin Invest* 1970;49:2172–87.

12. Oosterveer DM, Versmissen J, Yazdanpanah M et al. Differences in characteristics and risk of cardiovascular disease in familial hypercholesterolemia patients with and without tendon xanthomas: a systematic review and meta-analysis. *Atherosclerosis* 2009;207:311–17.

13. Silva PS, Gupta A, Ajlan RS et al. Ultrawide field scanning laser ophthalmoscopy imaging of lipemia retinalis. *Acta Ophthalmol* 2018; 96:e643–6.

14. Zahavi A, Snir M, Kella YR. Lipemia retinalis: case report and review of the literature. *J AAPOS* 2013;17:110–11.

15. Rymarz E, Matysik-Woźniak A, Baltaziak L et al. Lipemia retinalis – an unusual cause of visual acuity deterioration. *Med Sci Monit* 2012; 18:CS72–5.

16. Nordestgaard BG. Triglyceride-rich lipoproteins and atherosclerotic cardiovascular disease: new insights from epidemiology, genetics, and biology. *Circ Res* 2016;118:547–63.

17. Do R, Stitziel NO, Won H-H et al. Exome sequencing identifies rare LDLR and APOA5 alleles conferring risk for myocardial infarction. *Nature* 2015;518:102–6.

18. Ebara T, Endo Y, Yoshiike S et al. A 60-y-old chylomicronemia patient homozygous for missense mutation (G188E) in the lipoprotein lipase gene showed no accelerated atherosclerosis. *Clin Chim Acta* 2007;386:100–4.

19. Benes LB, Brandt EJ, Davidson MH. Advances in diagnosis and potential therapeutic options for familial chylomicronemia syndrome. *Expert Opin Orphan Drugs* 2018; 6:141–9.

20. Sniderman AD, Islam S, Yusuf S, McQueen MJ. Discordance analysis of apolipoprotein B and non-high density lipoprotein cholesterol as markers of cardiovascular risk in the INTERHEART study. *Atherosclerosis* 2012;225:444–9.

21. Benlian P, De Gennes JL, Foubert L et al. Premature atherosclerosis in patients with familial chylomicronemia caused by mutations in the lipoprotein lipase gene. *N Engl J Med* 1996;335:848–54.

4 Management and prevention

FCS is characterized by extreme hypertriglyceridemia, which causes physical, neurological and psychosocial symptoms (see Chapter 3), all of which need to be managed and, if possible, prevented. A summary of FCS management is provided in Table 4.1.

TABLE 4.1

Management of FCS

FCS population	Management recommendation
All populations	• Establish a multidisciplinary healthcare team to manage FCS and develop an individualized treatment plan
	• Eat a very-low-fat diet: <20 g fat per day or <10–15% daily caloric intake
	• Avoid alcohol
	• Avoid drugs known to increase TG levels
	• Measure plasma TG levels on a routine basis
Episodes of acute pancreatitis	• Hydrate patients with intravenous fluids
	• Once attack has subsided, slowly reintroduce very-low-fat diet
	• Consider insulin therapy in hyperglycemic patients
	• Some experts recommend a low threshold to initiate plasmapheresis or plasma exchange until serum TG is >5.65–11.3 mmol/L (500–1000 mg/dL); there are small risks associated with this, including transfusion reaction if plasma products are given back during plasma exchange

(CONTINUED)

TABLE 4.1 (CONTINUED)

Management of FCS

FCS population	Management recommendation
Diabetes	• Control blood sugar; insulin is usually necessary due to pancreatic insufficiency • Check levels of vitamins A, E, K and D regularly
Pregnancy	• Maintain fasting plasma TG levels at <5.65 mmol/L (500 mg/dL) • Limit fat intake to <2 g/day from weeks 13 to 40 of pregnancy • Use supplements to promote preferential intake of medium-chain fatty acids* • Maintain adequate hydration and electrolyte balance
Pregnancy and diabetes	• Control blood glucose and TG levels • Monitor TG levels weekly • Check for eruptive xanthomas and lipemia retinalis
Pediatrics	• Limit fat to <15% of total daily caloric intake • Use supplements to promote preferential intake of medium-chain TGs* • Feed infants (0–12 months) a low light-chain/high medium-chain fatty acid formula or skim and fortified expressed breast milk* • Transition 1–2 year olds to skim milk and age-appropriate low-fat solid foods • Monitor growth using age-appropriate charts • Re-evaluate diet at each developmental stage and adjust for age and growth
Psychosocial	• Psychological and nutritional counseling • Connect to support groups, patient organizations and websites for support and to maintain social connections

*Medium-chain TGs are metabolized through a chylomicron-independent pathway.[2]

The key goal of managing FCS is to maintain plasma TG levels below 11.3 mmol/L (1000 mg/dL).[1] Patients with FCS do not usually respond to standard lipid-lowering medications. A very-low-fat diet and regular exercise are therefore the mainstays of treatment.

In Europe, an antisense oligonucleotide (ASO) therapy to apo C-III has been licensed for the treatment of FCS (see Medical management below). Other therapies are in development (see Chapter 5).

Multidisciplinary healthcare team

The FCS healthcare team may include a lipidologist, pancreatologist/hepatologist, primary care physician, registered dietitian, psychologist and social worker. Other specialists may also be involved, depending on the patient's specific medical condition(s). For example, pregnant women with FCS will require the involvement of an obstetrician, pregnant women with both FCS and diabetes will require the involvement of an obstetrician and a diabetologist/endocrinologist, and patients with both FCS and diabetes ought to have the support of a diabetologist/endocrinologist and/or gastroenterologist. In the UK, patients with FCS may be seen at a lipid or inherited metabolic disease clinic that specializes in treating hyperlipidemia and hypertriglyceridemia.

Together, the FCS healthcare team should develop an individual treatment plan for each patient and decide how this information should be communicated to the patient. It is important that healthcare teams meet with the patient and family members to discuss all treatment options and answer questions. This ensures the patient understands the importance of their long-term TG monitoring and follow-up.

Dietary management

To maintain plasma TG levels below 11.3 mmol/L (1000 mg/dL), patients must follow a severely restricted low-fat diet consisting of less than 20 g of fat per day or 10–15% of total caloric intake (Table 4.2). In addition, patients with FCS need to avoid alcohol, which increases TG levels.

When fat is used in the diet, medium-chain TG oils are recommended (although they may be hard to obtain in some countries), as medium-chain TGs are metabolized through a

TABLE 4.2

Recommended diet for patients with FCS

Dietary recommendations	Foods to eat	Foods to avoid
• Daily fat intake 10–15% of total calories	• White fish, some seafood, poultry and lean cuts of meat	• Alcohol
• Eat fat-free or low-fat protein at each meal or snack	• Vegetables	• Simple sugars
• Limit total carbohydrates; limit simple carbohydrates	• Whole grains	• Fruit juices
• Eat small frequent meals and snacks	• Legumes/pulses	
• Increase water intake	• Fat-free milk	
• Supplement fat-soluble vitamins (A, D, E, K), as needed	• Fat-free low-sugar dairy products	
	• Fruit	
	• Water	

chylomicron-independent pathway,[2] resulting in lower chylomicron-TG levels.[3]

Even with strict adherence to a low-fat diet, which is critical for patients with FCS, 90% of patients with FCS still report symptoms.[4] Furthermore, 80% of patients report that this diet is very difficult to maintain long term.[4] It takes an extraordinary amount of meal planning, and social eating is especially challenging.

Deviations from the diet, such as eating dietary fat or consuming alcohol, can result in large fluctuations in serum TG levels that increase the risk of acute pancreatitis, even when patients have followed the restricted diet the majority of the time. These factors contribute to the decreased quality of life reported by patients with FCS.[5]

Physical activity

Regular exercise is important, as it can reduce body fat and TG levels.[6] In healthy adults, exercise has been shown to induce changes in blood perfusion and increase LPL in exercising muscles. This may therefore lead to increased interactions between chylomicrons and LPL, thus contributing to lower levels of chylomicron-TG[7] and lower plasma TGs.[8]

Medical management

Standard lipid-lowering medications such as omega-3 fatty acids (or their derivatives), statins and fibrates have a reduced to no effect in patients with FCS.[1] However, as most of these agents have a low side-effect profile it is reasonable to try them. If there is no improvement in TG levels then they should be discontinued. As discussed in Chapter 2, a 3-month trial of a lipid-lowering drug can be used diagnostically, with non-response confirming the possibility of FCS.

Volanesorsen was approved in Europe in 2019 for the treatment of adults with FCS.

Mechanism of action. Volanesorsen is an ASO that reduces the production of apo C-III, a well-known inhibitor of LPL (see Chapter 1). Human exome sequencing has found that mutations resulting in *APOC3* loss of function are associated with both lower serum TG levels and a decreased risk of coronary heart disease.[9] More recently, apo C-III has been found to raise serum TG by LPL-independent pathways, including inhibition of hepatic lipase, increased production of VLDL and decreased hepatic receptor-mediated uptake of TG-rich lipoproteins.[10,11] These mechanisms may even predominate over the initially discovered LPL-dependent pathway.

Efficacy. In the CS6 (APPROACH) Phase III study, the efficacy and safety of volanesorsen was evaluated in 66 adult patients with TG levels greater than 8.48 mmol/L (750 mg/dL) and clinical FCS. Patients were randomized to subcutaneous volanesorsen, 285 mg weekly, or placebo. The primary endpoint was met, with a 94% reduction (20.4 mmol/L [1804 mg/dL]) in TG at 3 months. In the volanesorsen group, TG levels were reduced by 53% at 6 months and 40% at 12 months. In total, 77% of patients receiving volanesorsen (versus 10% of patients receiving placebo) were classified as responders, achieving TG levels lower than 8.48 mmol/L (750 mg/dL).[12]

In the COMPASS trial, the efficacy and safety of volanesorsen was investigated in 113 patients with hypertriglyceridemia with fasting

TG levels greater than 5.65 mmol/L (500 mg/dL). The 7 patients with FCS had a baseline TG of 25.8±11.0 mmol/L (2280±973 mg/dL) and achieved a 73±14% TG reduction.[13]

Tolerability. In the APPROACH trial, acute pancreatitis and abdominal pain occurred in 36% of patients in the volanesorsen group and 39% of patients in the placebo group ($p=0.62$).[12] In a post hoc analysis of patients who had had at least two episodes of pancreatitis over the previous 5 years, prior rates of 24 events in 7 patients (volanesorsen) and 17 events in 4 patients (placebo) were reduced to zero events in those who received volanesorsen and 4 events in 3 patients who received placebo ($p=0.02$). Self-reported abdominal pain intensity was also reduced in the volanesorsen-treated patients. Pancreatitis events were reduced with volanesorsen therapy (0 vs 6; $p=0.01$) but 1 patient on volanesorsen had pancreatitis 3 months after the last dose.

Ongoing trial data. Data from an ongoing multicenter Phase III open-label extension (OLE) trial of patients treated with volanesorsen (comprised of patients from the APPROACH and COMPASS studies and a group of additionally recruited patients with FCS) have shown a reduction in pancreatitis events, with 1 event in a patient receiving volanesorsen compared with 9 events in 6 patients receiving placebo ($p=0.02$). Reductions in TG of 39% were maintained up to 18 months.[14]

A global retrospective study of a subset of 22 patients from the APPROACH-OLE phase (ReFOCUS study), reported improvements in disease burden after volanesorsen therapy (median 222 days). More patients (40%) reported effective management of FCS symptoms after 3 months of treatment compared with before (19%). Almost all reported that their symptoms were controlled with diet after treatment (90% vs 55% before treatment). The number of FCS symptoms was reduced after 3 months of treatment with volanesorsen (median 3.5 vs 6.5; $p<0.05$). Reductions were seen in physical (47%, $p=0.009$), emotional (47%; $p=0.007$) and cognitive manifestations (46%; $p=0.03$), but not in pancreatitis admissions. Patients also reported improvements in their personal, social and professional lives, with more patients reporting 'no interference' (23% vs 5%) and fewer patients reporting high levels of interference (37% vs 59%).[15] Overall, these data suggest an improvement in quality of life after treatment.

Most volanesorsen-treated patients (82%) experienced injection-site reactions, with most occurring early in treatment. Across all the above studies, 10 patients discontinued treatment for this reason. Serious adverse events were reported in 13% of patients receiving volanesorsen. Three events, including two reports of thrombocytopenia ($<25 \times 10^9$/L) and a report of serum sickness, were treatment related. In the ongoing APPROACH-OLE study, 13 patients (19%) reported a serious adverse event and treatment was discontinued due to severe thrombocytopenia in 4 patients. Antibodies to the drug were reported.

Drug avoidance. A number of drugs are known to increase TG levels and these should be avoided (Table 4.3).[1,6]

Long-term monitoring

Long-term monitoring consists of routine measurement of plasma TG levels, which some patients may be able to achieve on their own. In one study, patients with hypertriglyceridemia who used a home meter

---

TABLE 4.3

Medications that patients with FCS should avoid

- Hormones/endocrine drugs
  - Estrogen
- Oncologic drugs
  - Tamoxifen
  - Bexarotene
- Dermatology drugs
  - Retinoids (e.g. isotretinoin)
- CVD drugs
  - High-dose thiazide diuretics
  - High-dose beta-blockers

- Immune function modifiers
- Immunosuppressants
- Systemic steroids
- HIV protease inhibitors
- Mental health drugs
- Second-generation antipsychotics
  - Sertraline
- Lipid drugs
- Bile acid sequestrants
- Fish-oil supplements (non-pharmacological)

Adapted from Burnett et al. 2017 and Leaf 2008.[1,6]

to measure TGs before a main meal and 4 hours postprandially showed improved dietary adherence as a result of self-monitoring.[16]

Managing attacks

The concern regarding acute pancreatitis in FCS means that patients with the disorder who present with abdominal pain should be considered a medical emergency. During a pancreatitis attack, patients should be hydrated with intravenous fluids and receive no food by mouth. Some patients may require low-dose insulin to treat hyperglycemia and help lower TGs. Once the attack has subsided, food should be reintroduced slowly until the strict low-fat diet can be resumed.[6]

Fasting alone is often insufficient for significant TG clearance. In severe cases, plasmapheresis or plasma exchange may be considered for more rapid clearance of TGs.

Pancreatic insufficiency

Damage to the pancreas as a result of recurrent bouts of pancreatitis may cause pancreatogenic diabetes (type 3c diabetes).[17] It is therefore important to control blood sugar levels in order to lower serum TG levels and prevent diabetes-related medical complications. In addition to causing diabetes, pancreatic insufficiency can also impair the digestion and absorption of nutrients, including fat-soluble vitamins (vitamins A, E, K, D). The levels of these vitamins should be regularly monitored and supplements provided to avoid bone problems and other complications.

FCS in pregnancy

During pregnancy, patients with FCS are advised to maintain plasma TG levels below 5.65 mmol/L (500 mg/dL) by limiting fat intake to less than 2 g per day between weeks 13 and 40 of pregnancy (that is, the second and third trimesters). It is also important for pregnant women with FCS to maintain adequate hydration and electrolyte balance, and supplement their diet with medium-chain fatty acids.[1,18] Pharmacological omega-3 fatty acid preparations are often used in the management of this condition under specialist supervision. Monthly monitoring of plasma TG concentrations is recommended.[18]

Pregnant patients with both FCS and diabetes need to control their blood glucose and TG levels to ensure proper fetal development.

In these women, TG and glucose levels should be monitored weekly and patients should be checked for eruptive xanthomas, lipemia retinalis, hepatosplenomegaly and/or abdominal pain.

FCS in children

For children with FCS the goal is to maintain adequate growth, brain and cognitive development, and meet age-appropriate milestones while following a strict low-fat diet. In the pediatric population, fat should be limited to less than 15% of the total daily caloric intake to maintain plasma TG levels below 11.3 mmol/L (1000 mg/dL).[19] Fat intake should be adjusted to meet the requirements for essential fatty acids. Additional fat may be provided with medium-chain fatty acids to attain 10–15% of the daily caloric intake from fat.[19]

Infants with FCS (0–12 months) should be fed a low-fat/low light-chain TG/high medium-chain TG formula, or skimmed and fortified expressed breast milk that is supplemented with essential fatty acids, fat-soluble vitamins (A, D, E, K) and mineral supplements, as needed.[19] As appropriate, 1–2 year olds should be transitioned to skimmed milk and age-appropriate low-fat solid foods[19] with adequate protein consumption.[20]

All children with FCS should undergo regular physical examination and laboratory tests, with monitoring against age-appropriate growth charts.[21,22] Parents and caregivers should receive regular counseling and advice regarding the low-fat dietary requirements of FCS, meal planning, age-appropriate foods, transitioning to table foods, and adjusting to school, play dates and social engagements.

Management of psychosocial effects

FCS has a significant impact on the daily lives of patients and caregivers, including their psychosocial and emotional health, and reduces quality of life.[3,5] Many patients with FCS report anxiety, fear and worry about food and eating, developing symptoms and overall health[5] as well as a reduced ability to work (91%).[4,5] Only 22% of patients with FCS report being employed full time. Furthermore, FCS has been shown to affect career choice, with 85% of those in full-time employment choosing less-demanding careers with little travel because of the challenges and effects of the disorder.[5]

The extreme restrictions of the low-fat diet have been shown to affect patients' emotional health as well as their social interactions and activities with peers, colleagues and family members.[4]

The psychosocial effect of FCS can be managed with psychological and nutritional counseling. Receiving support from others with FCS can decrease a patient's sense of isolation and anxiety about the disorder and help to develop social connections that can improve their quality of life.[23,24] Members of the healthcare team should refer patients to specific FCS forums, patient websites and local organizations for support (see Useful resources). Support groups have been shown to have a positive impact on the quality of life of patients, their caregivers and families.[25]

Patient self-care

Empowering patients to develop their own eating plan[26] and to accept personal responsibility for the self-management of their condition and their food choices[27] may be accomplished with collaborative and patient-centered practices[28] and shared decision-making[26,27] with all members of the healthcare team. A psychologist can lead this effort and work with patients to cultivate their own internal motivation to follow a restricted low-fat diet.

Support groups will help patients and their caregivers discuss the challenges of the condition, find resources and develop social connections that can improve their lives.[23,24] Such social connections have a positive effect on quality of life,[25] improve overall health[29] and reduce stress.[30]

Genetic counseling

As discussed in Chapter 1, FCS is an autosomal recessive inherited disorder, so the children of patients with monogenic FCS have a 25% chance of being either affected or unaffected and a 50% chance of being an asymptomatic carrier of the disorder.[1] Genetic counseling is recommended for all at-risk family members of a person with FCS, especially if the genetic mutation has been identified. Genetic counseling can help the patient and family members better understand their condition, prevent the development of symptoms and other comorbid conditions, and use this information for family planning purposes.

Key points – management and prevention

- Management of FCS primarily involves following an extremely restricted low-fat diet (<20 g of fat per day or 10–15% of total caloric intake) and regular exercise.
- Patients with FCS should also limit their carbohydrate intake and avoid alcohol, simple sugars and drugs known to increase TG levels.
- Long-term monitoring consists of routine measurement of plasma TG levels.
- Given the risk of acute pancreatitis associated with FCS, patients with the condition who present with abdominal pain should be considered a medical emergency. Treatment should comprise intravenous fluids and withholding enteral nutrition, consideration of intravenous insulin for hyperglycemia, and plasmapheresis or plasma exchange in severe cases.
- Patients with FCS may develop pancreatogenic (type 3c) diabetes.
- During pregnancy, patients with FCS should be managed by specialist units and advised to maintain plasma TG levels below 5.65 mmol/L (500 mg/dL) by limiting fat intake to less than 2 g per day during the second and third trimesters. Pregnant women will need a lot of support to achieve this.
- Pregnant patients with FCS and diabetes need to control their blood glucose and TG levels, which should be monitored weekly.
- Infants with FCS should be fed a low-fat/low light-chain TG/ high medium-chain TG formula or skim and fortified expressed breast milk supplemented with essential fatty acids, fat-soluble vitamins (A, D, E, K) and mineral supplements.
- Children with FCS should limit dietary fat to less than 15% of total daily caloric intake to maintain plasma TG levels below 11.3 mmol/L (1000 mg/dL). Fat intake should be adjusted to meet the requirements for essential fatty acids.
- Support from patient organizations and websites will help patients and their caregivers to discuss challenges, find resources and develop social connections that can improve their lives and overall health.
- Genetic counseling is recommended for all newly diagnosed patients and their families.

References

1. Burnett JR, Hooper AJ, Hegele RA. Familial lipoprotein lipase deficiency. In: Adam MP, Ardinger HH, Pagon RA et al., eds. *GeneReviews®* [Internet]. Seattle, Washington: University of Washington, Seattle; 1993–2018. 1999 Oct 12 [updated 22 June 2017].

2. Bryant LM, Christopher DM, Giles AR et al. Lessons learned from the clinical development and market authorization of Glybera. *Human Gene Ther Clin Dev* 2013;24:55–64.

3. Hauenschild A, Bretzel RG, Schnell-Kretschmer H et al. Successful treatment of severe hypertriglyceridemia with a formula diet rich in omega-3 fatty acids and medium-chain fatty acids. *Ann Nutr Metab* 2010;56:170–5.

4. Gelrud A, Williams KR, Hsieh A et al. The burden of familial chylomicronemia syndrome from the patients' perspective. *Expert Rev Cardiovasc Ther* 2017;15:879–87.

5. Davidson M, Stevenson M, Hsieh A et al. The burden of familial chylomicronemia syndrome: interim results from the IN-FOCUS study. *Expert Rev Cardiovasc Ther* 2017;15: 415–23.

6. Leaf DA. Chylomicronemia and the chylomicronemia syndrome: a practical approach to management. *Am J Med* 2008;121:10–12.

7. Leaf DA, Parker DL, Schaad D. Changes in VO2max, physical activity, and body fat with chronic exercise: effects on plasma lipids. *Med Sci Sports Exerc* 1997;29:1152–9.

8. Enevoldsen LH, Simonsen L, Bulow J. Postprandial triacylglycerol uptake in the legs is increased during exercise and post-exercise recovery. *J Physiol* 2005;568:941–50.

9. Crosby J, Peloso GM, Auer PL et al.; TG and HDL Working Group of the Exome Sequencing Project, National Heart, Lung, and Blood Institute. Loss-of-function mutations in APOC3, triglycerides, and coronary disease. *N Engl J Med* 2014;371:22–31.

10. Yang X, Lee SR, Choi YS et al. Reduction in lipoprotein-associated apoC-III levels following volanesorsen therapy: phase 2 randomized trial results. *J Lipid Res* 2016;57:706–13.

11. Benes LB, Brandt EJ, Davidson MH. Advances in diagnosis and potential therapeutic options for familial chylomicronemia syndrome. *Expert Opin Orphan Drugs* 2018; 6:141–9.

12. Witztum JL, Gaudet D, Freedman SD et al. Volanesorsen and triglyceride levels in familial chylomicronemia syndrome. *N Engl J Med* 2019;381:531–42.

13. Gouni-Berthold I, Alexander V, Digenio A et al. Apolipoprotein C-III inhibition with volanesorsen in patients with hypertriglyceridemia (COMPASS): a randomized, double-blind, placebo-controlled trial. *Athero Suppl* 2017;28:e1–e2.

14. Gelrud A, Digenio A, Alexander V et al. Treatment with volanesorsen (VLN) reduced triglycerides and pancreatitis in patients with FCS and sHTG vs placebo: results of the APPROACH and COMPASS. *J Clin Lipidol* 2018;12:537.

15. Arca M, Hsieh A, Soran H et al. The effect of volanesorsen treatment on the burden associated with familial chylomicronemia syndrome: the results of the ReFOCUS study. *Expert Rev Cardiovasc Ther* 2018; 16:537–46.

16. Hauenschild A, Ewald N, Schnell-Kretschmer H et al. Successful long-term treatment of severe hypertriglyceridemia by feedback control with lipid self-monitoring. *Ann Nutr Metab* 2008;52:215–20.

17. Rickels MR, Bellin M, Toledo FGS et al. Detection, evaluation, and treatment of diabetes mellitus in chronic pancreatitis: recommendations from PancreasFest 2012. *Pancreatology* 2013;13:336–42.

18. Goldberg AS, Hegele RA. Severe hypertriglyceridemia in pregnancy. *J Clin Endocrinol Metab* 2012;97: 2589–96.

19. Williams L, Wilson DP. Editorial commentary: dietary management of familial chylomicronemia syndrome. *J Clin Lipidol* 2016;10:462–5.

20. Institute of Medicine. Food and Nutrition Board. *Dietary Reference Intakes for Energy, Carbohydrate, Fiber, Fat, Fatty Acids, Cholesterol, Protein, and Amino Acids (Macronutrients).* Washington, DC: National Academies Press, 2005.

21. Williams L, Rhodes KS, Karmally W et al. Familial chylomicronemia syndrome: bringing to life dietary recommendations throughout the life span. *J Clin Lipidol* 2018; 12:908–19.

22. National Center for Health Statistics. WHO growth standards are recommended for use in the U.S. for infants and children 0 to 2 years of age. Centers for Disease Control and Prevention. www.cdc.gov/ growthcharts/who_charts.htm, last accessed 11 June 2021.

23. Cruwys T, Alexander HS, Dingle GA et al. Feeling connected again: interventions that increase social identification reduce depression symptoms in community and clinical settings. *J Affect Disord* 2014;159: 139–46.

24. Wilson LM, Cross RR, Duell PB. Reduced psychologic distress in familial chylomicronemia syndrome after patient support group intervention. *J Clin Lipidol* 2018; 12:240–2.

25. House JS, Landis KR, Umberson D. Social relationships and health. *Science* 1988;241:540–5.

26. Snetselaar L. *Nutrition Counseling Skills for the Nutrition Care Process*, 4th edn. Sudbury, Massachusetts: Jones and Bartlett Publishers LLC, 2009:27.

27. Bodenheimer T, Lorig K, Holman H et al. Patient self-management of chronic disease in primary care. *JAMA* 2002;288:2469–75.

28. Funnell MM, Anderson RM. Empowerment and self-management of diabetes. *Clinical Diabetes* 2004; 22:123–7.

29. Rico-Uribe LA, Cabellero FF, Olaya B et al. Loneliness, social networks, and health: a cross-sectional study in three countries. *PLoS One* 2016;11:e0145264.

30. Kopp MS, Skrabski A, Szekeley A et al. Chronic stress and social changes: socioeconomic determination of social stress. *Ann NY Acad Sci* 2007;1113:325–38.

Natural history studies

The natural history of FCS has not been well described. The clinical course is likely to diverge with the development of pancreatitis because of the high morbidity and mortality associated with it. One episode of acute pancreatitis is usually the first of many, whereas a more normal life-course may be possible for those who never develop pancreatitis. Whether a patient with FCS is susceptible to abdominal pain and/or acute bouts of pancreatitis is largely dependent on serum TG levels, therefore the success of TG-lowering strategies is also a key factor in the natural history of the disorder.

Additional genetic factors also appear to influence each patient's propensity to develop recurrent bouts of acute pancreatitis. For example, those with a mutation/variant in the *CFTR* gene have an increased risk of developing acute pancreatitis in the setting of severe hypertriglyceridemia.[1]

Severely elevated serum TG levels also cause eruptive xanthomas, hepatosplenomegaly and/or neurocognitive dysfunction in the absence of pancreatitis (see Chapter 3). Therefore, serum TG control or the presence of pancreatitis alone cannot predict the clinical course, and both are likely to need factoring in when trying to predict prognosis.

Further study of the natural history of FCS would identify more specific factors that affect prognosis and would determine the effect of successful TG-lowering interventions in terms of future morbidity and life expectancy. To maximize the use of expensive preventive medication, factors enabling us to predict susceptibility to pancreatitis are urgently needed. The GENIALL database (Gene Therapy in the Management of Lipoprotein Lipase Deficiency) was created in 2014 to follow the natural history of patients with LPL deficiency, including those who received gene therapy with alipogene tiparvovec (see below).[2] While this only represents one subtype of FCS, this study is likely to provide significant insights into the condition. A registry database enrolling any patient with FCS will be helpful, as it may offer useful comparisons between monogenic and polygenic forms of the disorder.

Understanding the burden of FCS

While several reports have discussed the physical manifestations and complications of FCS, assessments of the psychological burden are sparse. The first major report to describe the psychological and neurocognitive effects of FCS was the previously described IN-FOCUS internet-based survey (Investigation of Findings and Observations Captured in Burden of Illness Survey). It found that about one-third of patients with FCS experience psychological morbidity.[3] At the time of publication, 166 patients with FCS from around the world had completed the survey and more continue to be enrolled. IN-FOCUS has been immensely helpful, but it is limited by the fact that it contains self-reported data; objectively measured data on this topic are lacking. Additional studies that objectively quantify both the prevalence of physical manifestations and the burden of FCS are needed.

The socioeconomic cost. Many patients with FCS need frequent hospitalization for recurrent bouts of acute pancreatitis, which adds burden to healthcare systems. In a study of patients with FCS who had a history of acute pancreatitis, the number of self-reported episodes ranged from 6 to 60, with a median of 17 episodes requiring hospitalization.[4] (Of note, a selection bias for sicker patients was likely to have occurred in this study, since 100% of the patients had a history of pancreatitis. The actual prevalence appears to be closer to 40–60%.) In the USA, the estimated cost of one hospitalization for acute pancreatitis is $31 820.[5]

The need for frequent hospitalizations can have a devastating impact on job opportunities and income. Many people with FCS report pursuing a career that accommodates their diagnosis, which can greatly limit their employment options and income. At present, managing FCS results in significant societal costs, but this is in part due to the absence of effective treatment options. Additional cost analyses of the healthcare burden for managing these patients are needed. This would, in part, help to determine which of the expensive potential future treatment options might be the most cost-effective despite the high baseline treatment expense.

Development of new therapies

Next-generation ASOs. Tolerability has been noted to be a problem with ASOs and a new liver-targeted technology based on high first-pass liver extraction (through the asialoglycoprotein receptor) of modified small interfering RNA molecules may allow doses of active agents to be reduced while preserving efficacy and reducing adverse events. AKCEA-APOCIII-LRx is a ligand-conjugated antisense drug comprising an ASO to apo C-III with an *N*-acetylgalactosamine-containing adduct to increase first-pass hepatic clearance. In a multiple-dose study, patients received 15 mg and 30 mg weekly or 60 mg every 4 weeks and achieved TG reductions of 59%, 73% and 66%, respectively.[6] A trial of AKCEA-APOCIII-LRx (ISIS 678354) for reduction of TGs in patients with hypertriglyceridemia is under way.

Lipoprotein lipase gene therapy. As most patients with FCS have either defective or deficient LPL activity, or deficient transport of LPL to the endothelial surface, it would be ideal if they could be given an LPL replacement. However, LPL has a short half-life, so this has not yet been feasible. Gene therapy with alipogene tiparvovec, on the other hand, was a potential means of circumventing the inability to administer a normal LPL replacement protein.

Alipogene tiparvovec encodes a naturally occurring gain-of-function variant of *LPL* carried by an adeno-associated virus vector.[7] Study results showed that after intramuscular injection it was incorporated into the host DNA and subsequently led to transcription of the gain-of-function *LPL*. Interestingly, although 2-year follow-up revealed a return to baseline TG levels, there was still a reduction in the occurrence of acute pancreatitis.[8] Patients with FCS who were followed up for 6 years showed a reduction in episodes of acute pancreatitis, abdominal pain and the number of hospitalizations.[7]

Although alipogene tiparvovec was an effective treatment option, its high cost and low demand meant that it was only administered to one patient in the clinical setting, and it was withdrawn from the market in 2017.

Angiopoietin-like protein 3 inhibition. Although the functions of angiopoietin-like protein 3 (ANGPTL3) and related angiopoietin-like proteins are not fully known at this time, in addition to promoting angiogenesis they appear to inhibit LPL. Inhibition of ANGPTL3 has been shown to lower LDL-cholesterol, and therapy that targets ANGPTL3 is now being investigated as a treatment for familial hypercholesterolemia.

ANGPTL3 was first discovered in 2002: genome-wide association studies and exome-sequencing studies found reduced levels of both TG and LDL-cholesterol in those with genetic loss-of-function variants of *ANGPTL3* or *ANGPTL4*. Furthermore, individuals with loss-of-function variants of *ANGPTL3* had a lower risk of atherosclerotic CVD.[9]

Evinacumab is a fully humanized monoclonal antibody that targets ANGPTL3. In one study, evinacumab reduced fasting TG and LDL-cholesterol by as much as 76% and 23%, respectively, in humans with mild-to-moderate hypertriglyceridemia.[9] There were no significant safety concerns.

Evinacumab is being studied in the FCS population as it is hypothesized to show greater benefit in individuals with some functional LPL activity and as there appear to be other LPL-independent mechanisms of TG lowering. As more is discovered about ANGPTL4, ANGPTL8 and other ANGPTLs, they may become future treatment targets for TG lowering.

Key points – research directions

- Serum TG levels and the propensity to develop recurrent bouts of acute pancreatitis are likely to affect the course of the disorder and prognosis in patients with FCS. More natural history studies are needed to help determine prognostic factors.
- Any database that enrolls patients with FCS provides helpful insights into the condition and may offer better comparisons between monogenic and polygenic forms of FCS. At present, the IN-FOCUS and GENIALL databases are helpful in determining the course of the disorder.
- The average cost of hospitalization for one episode of acute pancreatitis in the USA is $31 820. Cost analyses may reveal that targeted therapies for FCS are more cost-effective than previously realized.
- Future drug therapies for FCS include inhibitors of apo C-III and angiopoietin-like proteins.
- Future research on the healthcare costs of FCS may reopen the door for *LPL* gene therapy.

References

1. Valdivielso P, Ramírez-Bueno A, Ewald N. Current knowledge of hypertriglyceridemic pancreatitis. *Eur J Intern Med* 2014;25:689–94.

2. Steinhagen-Thiessen E, Stroes E, Soran H et al.; GENIALL investigators. The role of registries in rare genetic lipid disorders: review and introduction of the first global registry in lipoprotein lipase deficiency. *Atherosclerosis* 2017; 262:146–53.

3. Davidson M, Stevenson M, Hsieh A et al. The burden of familial chylomicronemia syndrome: interim results from the IN-FOCUS study. *Expert Rev Cardiovasc Ther* 2017; 15:415–23.

4. Gelrud A, Williams KR, Hsieh A et al. The burden of familial chylomicronemia syndrome from the patients' perspective. *Expert Rev Cardiovasc Ther* 2017;15:879–87.

5. Gaudet D, Signorovitch J, Swallow E et al. Medical resource use and costs associated with chylomicronemia. *J Med Econ* 2013;16:657–66.

6. Alexander VJ, Xia S, Hurh E et al. *N*-acetyl galactosamine-conjugated antisense drug to APOC3 mRNA, triglycerides and atherogenic lipoprotein levels. *Eur Heart J* 2019;40:2785–96.

7. Gaudet D, Stroes ES, Méthot J et al. Long-term retrospective analysis of gene therapy with alipogene tiparvovec and its effect on lipoprotein lipase deficiency-induced pancreatitis. *Hum Gene Ther* 2016; 27:916–25.

8. Gaudet D, Méthot J, Déry S et al. Efficacy and long-term safety of alipogene tiparvovec (AAV1-LPLS447X) gene therapy for lipoprotein lipase deficiency: an open-label trial. *Gene Ther* 2013;20:361–9.

9. Dewey FE, Gusarova V, Dunbar RL et al. Genetic and pharmacologic inactivation of ANGPTL3 and cardiovascular disease. *N Engl J Med* 2017;377:211–21.

Useful resources

Action FCS
www.facebook.com/ActionFCS
www.actionfcs.org

EURODIS – Rare Diseases Europe
www.eurodis.org

FCS Focus
www.facebook.com/fcsfocus/
fcsfocus.com

FCS Foundation
www.facebook.com/fightFCS
www.livingwithfcs.org

FCS Rare Disease Report
fcs.raredr.com

GUTS UK
www.gutscharity.org.uk

Heart UK
www.heartuk.org.uk

National Organization for Rare Disorders (USA)
www.rarediseases.org/physician-guide
/lipoprotein-lipase-deficiency-lpld
www.rarediseases.org/rare-diseases
/familial-lipoprotein-lipase-deficiency

National Pancreas Foundation (USA)
www.pancreasfoundation.org/patient
-information/ailments-pancreas/familial
-chylomicronemia-syndrome

Index